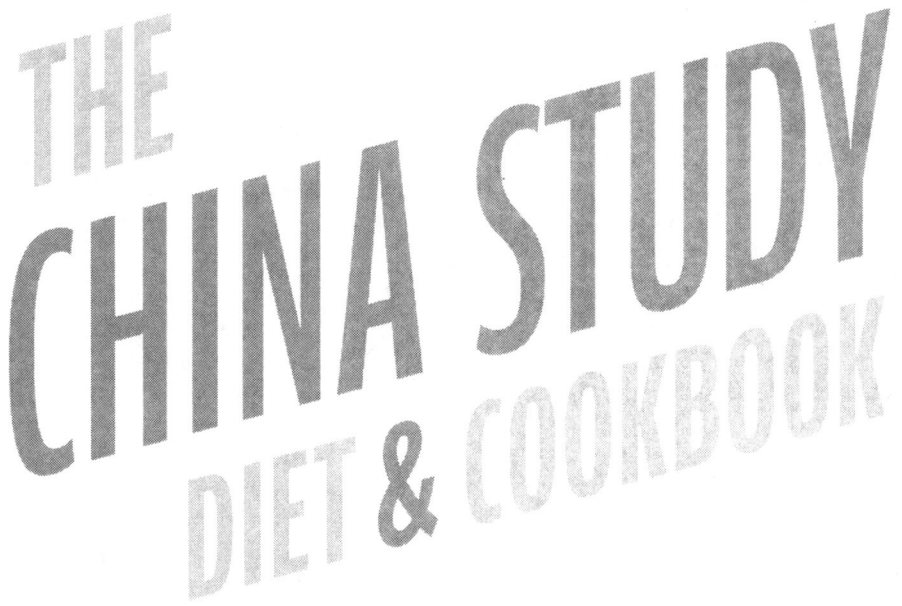

THE CHINA STUDY DIET & COOKBOOK

75 Essential **Plant-Based Recipes**
to **Lose Weight** and **Improve Health**

Rockridge Press

TABLE OF CONTENTS

INTRODUCTION

Hello and thank you for choosing this book to learn about the China Study and the diet that sprang forth from it. If you're reading this, you're probably interested in getting healthy or losing weight, or perhaps a little bit of both. If so, you're on the right track. Let us start with a bit of clarification: the China Study Diet isn't actually a diet. It's a lifestyle that results from the desire to be healthy. There's not an ideology or philosophy attached to it—there are no religious connotations—and there are only a couple of set-in-stone rules. It's simply a map to better health based upon scientific research.

Choosing the "Right" Healthy Path

Public interest in health is at an all-time high but so, unfortunately, is the popularity of baseless diets that lure the eager down a path that often leads to failure. You can't turn on the TV or flip through a magazine without seeing ads that promise to make you healthier, thinner, or more attractive.

Newsflash: Most of those ads are just bunk. There is no such thing as a quick fix—it takes dedication and commitment to follow a healthy lifestyle that leads to lifelong good health and weight loss. There is just so much information, both good and bad, that it's hard to choose exactly which plan to follow.

Sometimes one of the easiest ways to determine the merits of a diet is to take a close look at what it promises and what it requires. If a plan promises that you'll lose twenty-five pounds in three weeks or that it will eliminate disease from your body, it's probably quackery or extremely dangerous.

If a diet requires a huge, restrictive change in the way that you eat, or encourages you to eat mass amounts of just a handful of foods or vitamins, chances are good that it's unhealthy. In addition, you're not likely to stick to a diet that severely restricts what you can eat long-term, so you're ultimately not going to be successful.

That being said, if you're currently subsisting on donuts, pizza, and coffee, you're going to need to make massive changes in the way that you eat if you want to thrive for long. Don't worry though. We're going to show you how you can make the change that leads to lifelong health without counting calories, losing flavor, or limiting yourself to just a few foods. What you will lose is excess weight, points off of your cholesterol, and a myriad of other disease-causing conditions that are just time bombs waiting to make you sick.

So What Exactly Is the China Study?

The China Study, conducted by T. Colin Campbell, PhD, jointly with Cornell University and the Chinese Academy of Preventive Medicine, is the most comprehensive, longest-running health and nutrition study in medical history. It's a thirty-plus-year-long, ongoing longitudinal study of the eating habits of 6,500 Chinese men living in 650 rural villages. The study examined the instances of forty-eight different types of cancer and other serious diseases.

The men who were the subjects of the China Study ate almost an entirely plant-based diet, with the occasional serving of fish. Instead of the malnutrition and poor health that was anticipated, the study revealed that these men were much healthier than their

American counterparts. There were very few instances of cancer, heart disease, diabetes, and other "diseases of affluence." As a matter of fact, in the villages where the diet was entirely plant-based, these diseases were practically nonexistent.

The results of the study were startling to say the least. So startling, in fact, that Dr. Campbell was compelled to make his results public in an attempt to redefine what Western civilization considers good nutrition and healthful eating habits. One of the ways that he attempted to present and distribute his findings was via his book, *The China Study*.

Throughout the following chapters, we'll discuss how the China Study Diet can help you get healthy, and why the typical Western diet is killing us. We'll also talk about why it's taken so long for the concept of plant-based eating to reach the light of day. Finally, we'll share some great recipes that are so tasty that you'll never know that you're being good.

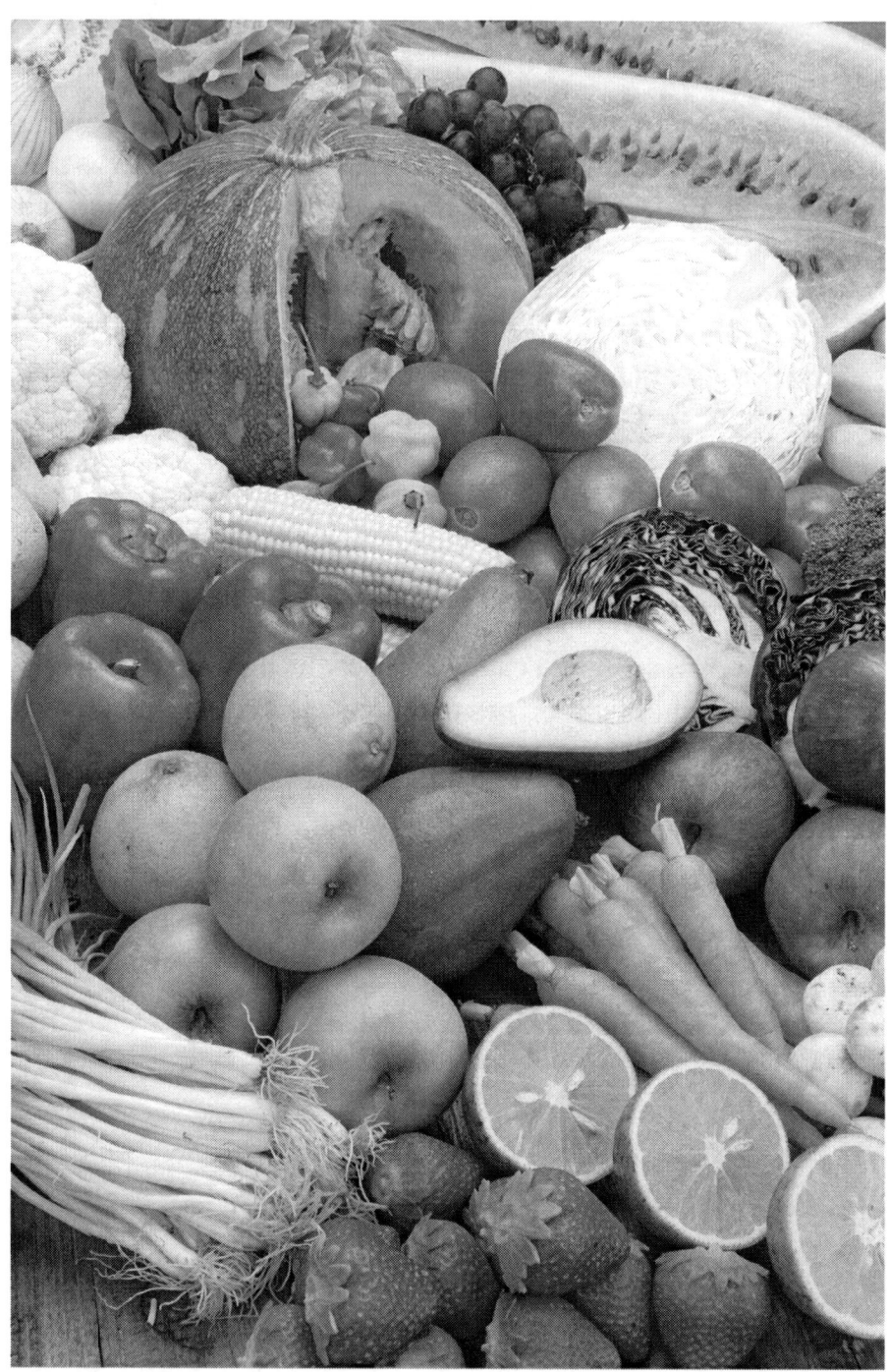

Plant-based diets are proven disease fighters and contribute to healthy weight management and overall well-being.

PART 1

The China Study Diet Demystified

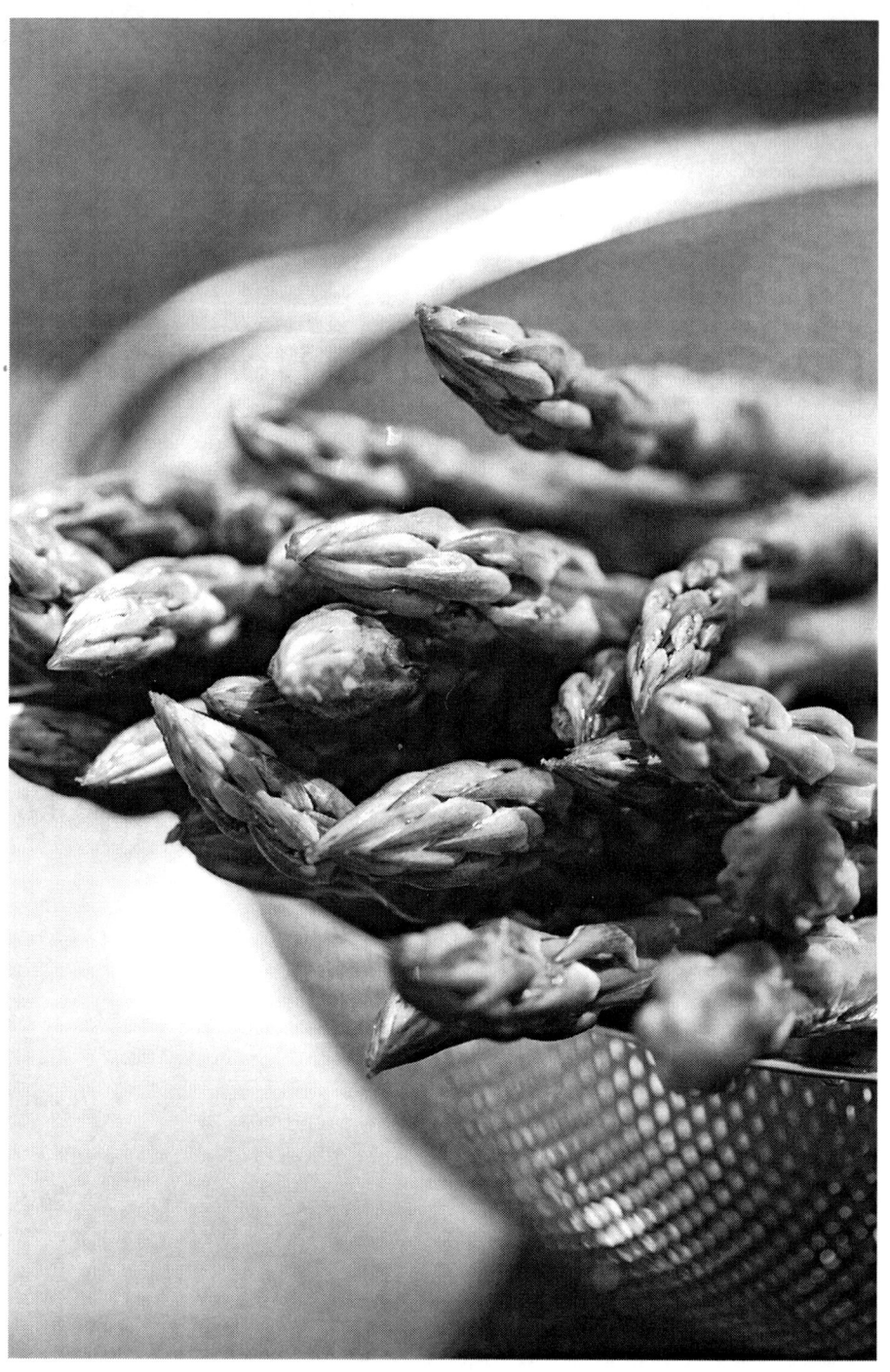

Asparagus has a sweet, nutty flavor and works well as a side dish for almost any meal.

1

DISEASES OF AFFLUENCE

For decades, and even centuries, Western doctors have promoted a diet high in protein and low in fat and calories. In particular, animal protein is considered to be far superior to plant protein and is the form most encouraged by Western doctors. This is an old-school way of thinking and has been proven incorrect by modern research.

As a matter of fact, there are numerous studies that have been conducted comparing the Western way of eating to the dietary traditions of other cultures. Almost invariably, people who eat Western-style are sicker, fatter, and more prone to disease than any other humans on the planet.

Don't Blame It on Genetics

When people develop diabetes, heart disease, cancer, or other illnesses, there's a huge tendency to blame it on genetics. Indeed, there are certain people who are predisposed to such conditions because of family history, but it's not always a given that just because Great Aunt Grace was diabetic, you will be too.

The more we learn about DNA and genetic proclivities, the more we understand that, in the vast majority of cases, behavioral decisions such as diet and exercise play a much larger role in the development of diseases than genetics do. You see, even though you may have the genes that increase your chances for cancer or diabetes, if they're never triggered, then those diseases do not become active.

Let's use diabetes as an example. If you stuff yourself full of refined sugar on a regular basis for long periods of time, and your body is genetically predisposed to develop insulin resistance, then you've created an environment in which it will. You've just unlocked your genetic predisposition to be diabetic. If you follow a diet low in refined sugars and high in complex carbohydrates locked in fiber that naturally regulates the release of glucose into your bloodstream, then you're setting the scene to leave those genes locked up forever. It's a choice that you make.

What Are Diseases of Affluence?

It seems logical that as people become wealthier, they can afford better foods and will be healthier than their poorer counterparts. Apparently, logic has no part in it because, at least in Western society, people with means are actually more prone to developing heart disease, metabolic syndrome, diabetes, and other conditions brought about by poor diet.

Rich sauces, nutritionally poor breads, processed foods, and quick-order chain restaurants make it simple and cheap to eat poorly. In a rush? Pull into the drive-thru and grab a burger and fries. Don't feel like cooking dinner? Toss a frozen meal in the microwave. It takes time and effort to cook a proper meal or plan ahead for a nutritious lunch, and people who can afford the convenient way out too often take it. And it's killing them.

As we drift further away from whole, natural foods, specifically plants, our food is instead laden with chemicals, sodium, and preservatives that provide very little nutrition and a whole lot of trans fats, cholesterol, and empty calories. Though we're eating twice what we should in calories, we're not getting nearly what we need to nourish our bodies and, as a society, we're getting sicker by the dollar.

In the China Study, there were very few instances of any of these disorders:

- Alzheimer's disease
- Cognitive impairment
- Heart disease
- Cancer
- Diabetes
- Metabolic syndrome
- Osteoporosis
- Obesity

Specifically, there is a group of diseases, including those listed, that have come to be known as "diseases of affluence," because they almost exclusively afflict prosperous societies that have adopted these less-than-healthy eating and lifestyle habits.

Let's take a look at some of these conditions, discuss what causes them, and talk about how plant-based nutrition can help you avoid or even reverse them.

Heart Disease

This is the biggest condition caused by poor eating, and is almost entirely avoidable simply by following a plant-based diet. As a matter of fact, the China Study revealed that in the villages that consumed a near-100 percent plant-based diet, not a single person was reported to have died from heart disease. That's pretty profound, but what's the connection?

What most people apparently don't realize is that when you're eating animal protein, you're also getting high amounts of LDL (bad) cholesterol with practically no HDL (good) cholesterol to level it out and keep it from wreaking havoc within your system.

You may not realize that cholesterol, in and of itself, isn't a bad thing. As a matter of fact, your body makes it. It's necessary in certain amounts in order to transport fat-soluble vitamins throughout your body, but when you eat too many saturated fats with the long-chain triglycerides that your body converts to LDL, the extra cholesterol begins to stick to the walls of your arteries and cause the plaque buildup, called atherosclerosis, that leads to heart disease.

These types of saturated fats are almost exclusively found in meats. Plant sources of saturated fat, such as coconut oil, consist of medium-chain triglycerides (MCTs) that your body converts mostly to energy instead of breaking it down into cholesterol. These MCTs also raise the "good" levels of cholesterol along with the "bad" ones, keeping them in balance.

Finally, plant-based fats such as coconut oil and avocado oil, as well as fresh fruits and vegetables, are rich in antioxidants that fight the free radicals that cause atherosclerosis and other damage to your cardiovascular system. Fiber found in grains and produce also helps to keep your system clean and running well.

There is documented data that shows that switching to a plant-based diet can actually reverse heart disease, at least to a certain degree. Plus, cutting out animal products and processed foods eliminates the cause of the plaque buildup, so making the switch is a win in several different ways.

Interestingly enough, most of the world's population who lead healthful lifestyles that include a plant-based diet and plenty of exercise are essentially free from heart disease. It is, indeed, a Western condition.

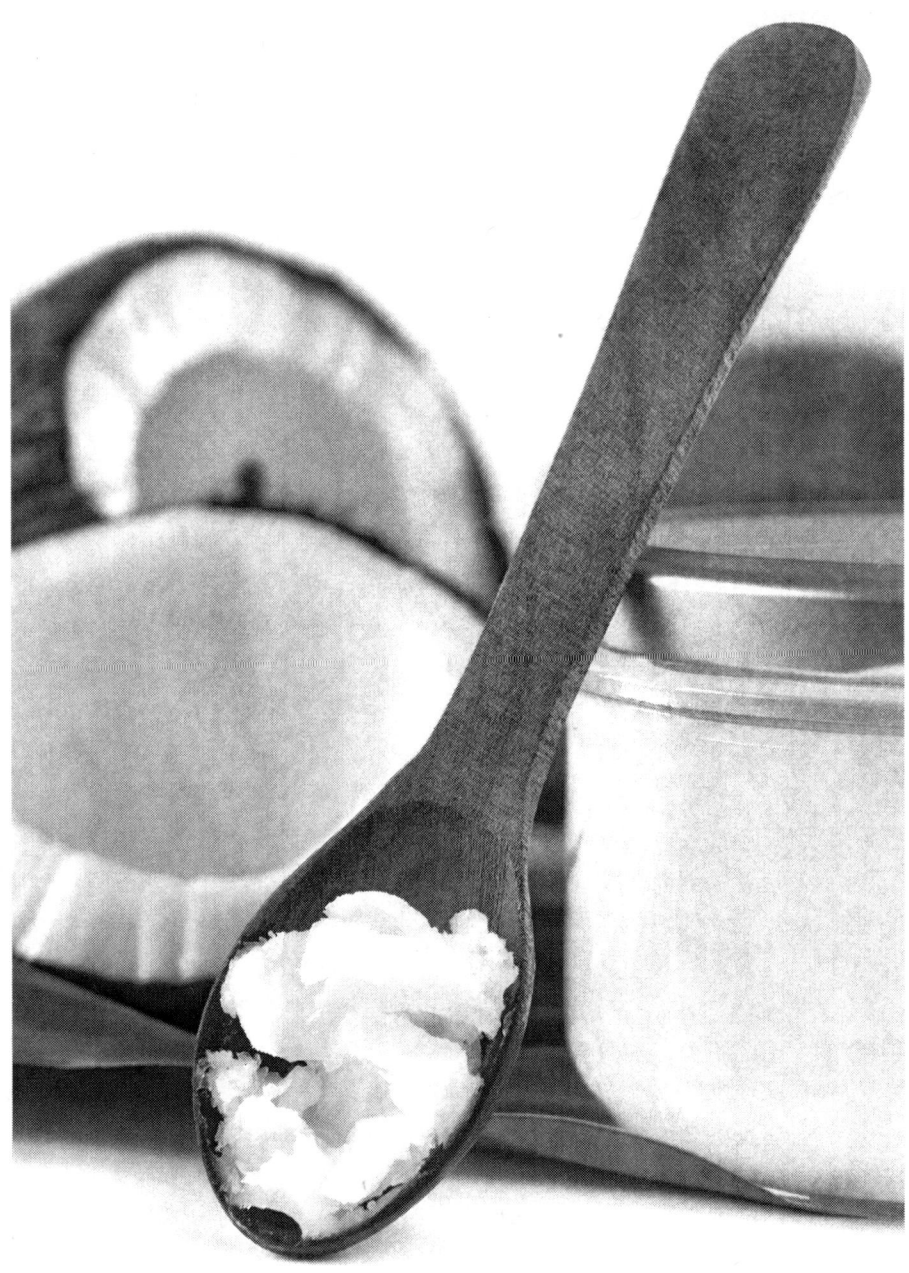

Plant sources of saturated fat, such as coconut oil, consist of medium-chain triglycerides that your body converts mostly to energy.

Diabetes

Many people believe that this is a genetic disorder that you're bound to get if your parents have it, but that's simply not true. Though you may be more inclined to develop diabetes than the person standing next to you, whether you activate those genes or not is largely dependent upon your lifestyle choices. As we learn more about insulin resistance in the human body, it becomes more obvious that type 2 diabetes is almost always avoidable simply by eating right and exercising.

In a nutshell, your body releases insulin when it gets the message that there's glucose (sugar) in the blood that needs to be picked up for conversion and transportation. When there's too much sugar on a regular basis, your body stops responding to the messages, and no insulin is released. At that point, the levels of glucose in your blood become dangerously high, causing all kinds of problems. It can be lethal if not controlled.

Simple carbohydrates are digested quickly, and sugar is released almost immediately into the bloodstream. That's why people who are in danger of passing out from low blood sugar may eat a piece of candy or even a pack of sugar; it takes only a few minutes for your body to break it down and throw it into your blood as glucose. As you can see, this can be a bad thing if done regularly and in large amounts.

Complex carbohydrates like those found in fruits and vegetables must be extracted from the fiber that's present in the produce. This is a much longer digestive process that releases glucose slowly into your system in smaller amounts. The difference between simple and complex carbohydrates is sort of like the difference between a blast from a water hose and a slow trickle at the sink; you may be releasing the same amount of water, but the trickle releases it in a steady, manageable amount.

There are no simple carbohydrates in a whole, plant-based diet so you never have to worry about making your body insulin-resistant. Type 2 diabetes is, for the most part, off the table as long as you eat responsibly.

Alzheimer's Disease

Your brain is made up largely of fatty acids, but in Alzheimer's patients, there is a mystery protein found in the brain that causes plaque to form. This causes cognitive decline and eventually other disorders, including Alzheimer's disease. Research has now positively linked Alzheimer's disease to insulin resistance; in fact, it's been classified as type 3 diabetes.

Since we already know what a diet full of simple sugars and starches does to exacerbate diabetes, we don't need to go on about what this implies. We'll just say that switching to a plant-based diet and avoiding plaque-causing substances found in animal proteins as well as simple sugars found in processed foods can help keep your brain healthy.

Cancer

Here it is: the big "C." If you ask people what they're most scared of dying from, this is the answer that you're going to get 90 percent of the time, and that fear is justified. An American man has about a 47 percent chance of getting cancer in his lifetime, according to the American Cancer Society.

Cancer is a debilitating disease that strips you of your dignity and leaves you begging for death. It's also one of the most researched diseases in the history of medicine, and, thanks to that research, we now know that it's largely preventable or even curable by eating a low-fat, low-protein, plant-based diet.

Free radicals caused by environmental toxins, bodily functions, and many other conditions cause a cell to mutate into something that is harmful to your body. This may manifest as damaged skin, heart disease, cancer, or a number of other conditions often related to aging or simply being human. There's good news, though.

Antioxidants in plants neutralize, and in some cases even destroy, free radicals that cause cancer. There is even a growing mountain of research showing that certain antioxidants can actually kill cancer cells in some instances. Another motivating factor to switch to a plant-based diet is that animal fats and proteins, as well as hormones that are often in them, play a huge role in many of the risk factors related to developing these types of cancer.

A great example of this is the female hormone estrogen, which is often added to meat or to animal feed. Studies indicate that even a 17 percent increase in estrogen levels in the body has a huge effect on breast cancer rates, so it only makes sense that if you eat a diet that's not adding estrogen to your body, your risk of breast cancer will be lower.

Dr. Campbell has actually dedicated a large portion of his life to researching cancer, and perhaps some of the most significant findings of the China Study relate to this vicious disease. He comments specifically on breast cancer, prostate cancer, and large bowel cancer in *The China Study*.

These are three types of cancer that are particularly affected by nutrition. As a matter of fact, what you eat is quite possibly the biggest factor in determining whether or not you're going to develop these cancers. Simply switching to a plant-based, low-protein diet rich in antioxidants can significantly decrease your odds of developing these and many other forms of cancer.

Obesity

It's not big news that cutting back on simple sugars and animal fats will cause you to lose weight. Perhaps the bigger issues are the diseases that are associated with obesity. Heart disease, diabetes, stroke, and just about every other health problem that can kill you is linked to obesity. The more obese you are, the greater your odds of developing other life-threatening conditions.

What may not be immediately obvious are a couple of other observations made while conducting the China Study. People who live on a low-fat, plant-based diet are not only prone to avoid obesity, but they also have more energy and are naturally more active.

Finally, people who depend upon animal sources for protein often take in significantly more calories than their plant-eating counterparts, and get less nutrition per spoonful. Combine this with the fact that they exercise less, and the path to obesity suddenly becomes a slippery slope. Don't turn to quick-fix diets or pills to lose weight; instead, change what's actually causing obesity: your diet and exercise habits.

These aren't all of the diseases associated with a life of plenty, either. Some others include:

- Leukemia
- Eye diseases
- Kidney stones
- Osteoporosis
- Stroke

Why Hasn't the China Study Diet Gone Mainstream?

The initial China Study was conducted from 1983 to 2003, and the results were indisputable and startling. So much so that it inspired Dr. Campbell to write a book and speak at functions about his work.

You may be asking yourself, though, why hasn't this already had a profound impact on the way that the public is instructed to eat? It's an excellent question and one that has some difficult answers.

Habit and Tradition

First and foremost, the animal-based diet has, for centuries, been the ideal for healthful eating. The need for protein to build lean muscle and carbohydrates for energy has been so ingrained into our collective psyches that it's difficult to make a change. The idea of a plate full of vegetables with no meat on the side just seems incomplete; without a steak or a piece of chicken, it just isn't a real meal. Old habits and social mores are hard to change.

Too Many "Diets" Crying Wolf

Remember all of those fads and fraud diets that we mentioned earlier? They've made it more difficult to get the idea of switching to a plant-based diet serious attention. Many people think that it's just a passing fad, even when the research is right there staring you in the face. Unfortunately, the China Study has largely become buried in a sea of quackery and misinformation.

Economics

Whenever you start messing with a person's livelihood, there are going to be issues, and there are quite literally billions of people whose livelihoods depend upon animal-based food supplies. If everyone were to immediately stop eating meat or other animal products, the economy would plummet, animals would be running amok, and chaos would ensue.

Politics

Beef is a big business, without a doubt. So are the poultry, egg, milk, cheese, and drug industries, and they don't take kindly to somebody strolling in and showing the American people research that indicates that they may be better off if they were to skip the animal products. These industries are powerful and swing a wide ax in political circles.

It's difficult to get government agencies to promote a change that may result in funding cuts and loss of revenue, and that's exactly what the FDA, USDA, and other government agencies are facing by promoting a plant-based diet as a healthful alternative to eating animal products.

All of these factors, plus some others, have combined to make it difficult for Dr. Campbell to effectively reach consumers on a large scale. His book has helped get the word out and so has the public's drive for healthier alternatives. As people educate themselves, plant-based nutrition is gaining popularity, but it hasn't been an easy road.

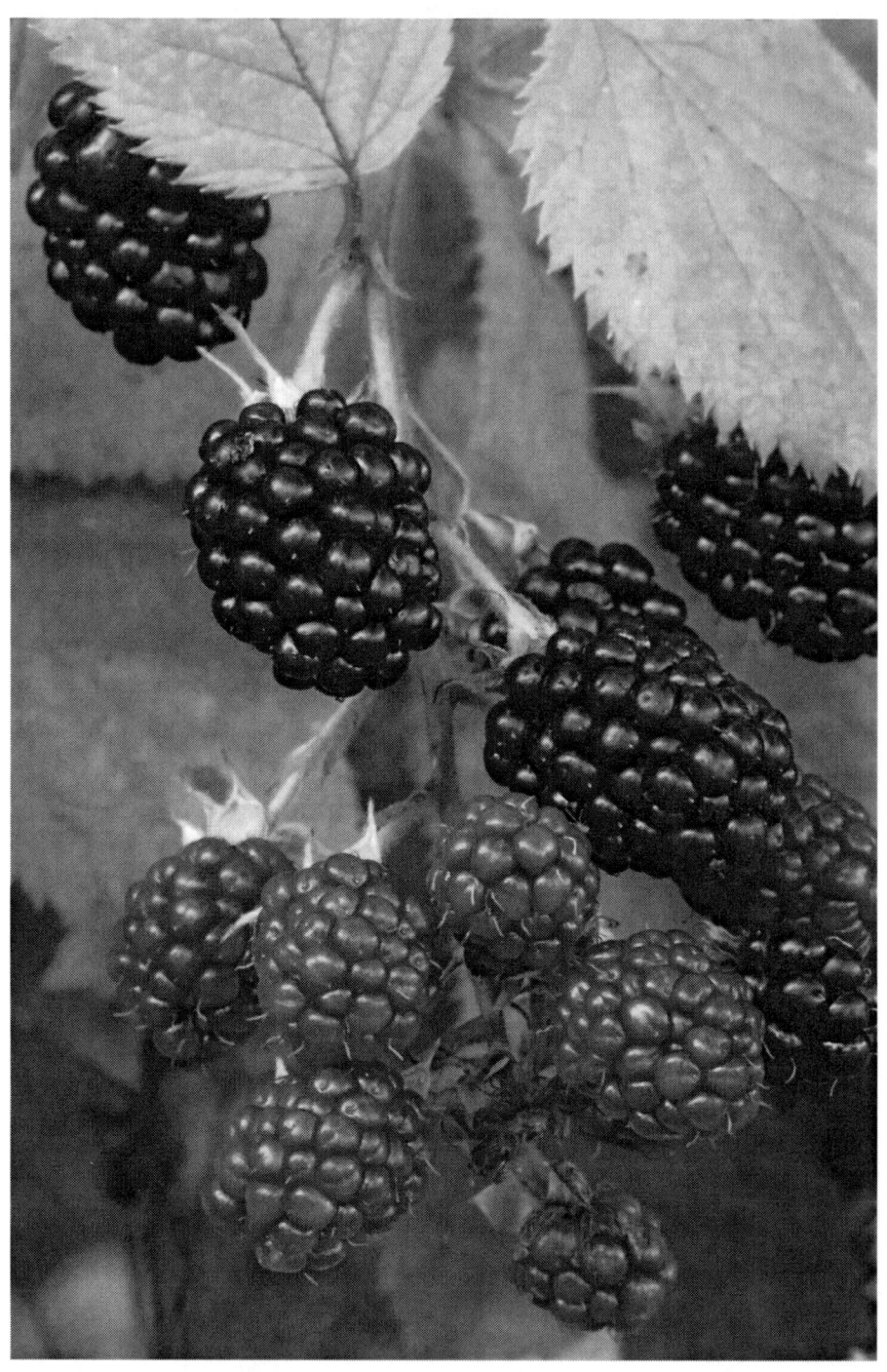

Blackberries are low in calories and very nutritious compared to other berries.

2

THE CHINA STUDY: EAST

D r. T. Colin Campbell wrote *The China Study* because he believed
that the American people needed to know the truth about what
was causing the rampant increase in death and disease in the United
States. He wanted to spread the word about what he discovered
during a lifetime of research. Most importantly, he wanted people
to know that the solution was simple and inexpensive. You can
effectively avoid and even reverse or eliminate most of the diseases
that are so prevalent in American society today.

As a typical Midwestern American raised on a dairy farm, Dr.
Campbell didn't start out as an advocate of animal-free eating. He
was a meat eater just like everybody around him, but as he began
to research the diseases and learn about the effects of nutrition on
the body, he slowly began to suspect that plant-based eating was a
natural preventive measure for many of the diseases that are killing
millions today.

In 1988, Dr. Campbell was asked to go before the U.S. Senate
Governmental Affairs Committee to explain why he thought that the
American public was so confused about nutrition and wellness. He
believed that it was because science became too focused on single
aspects of health such as the effects of one vitamin or one food on
nutrition without looking at the bigger picture.

That's exactly why his research was so diverse; he has studied many different types of diseases in different people and test animals under varied conditions. One of the most exciting findings was that he could actually turn cancer on and off by modifying the diet in lab animals, and the same results appear over and over again in humans too. The link between nutrition and health simply can't be denied.

The China Study was part of a diverse group of research studies and was conducted in China and Taiwan. Over a period of thirty-five years, Dr. Campbell and his associates completed seventy-five grant years' worth of work studying the link between disease and dietary practices. He was slowly but surely convinced by empirical evidence that the path to disease-free living lay in a plant-based diet and active lifestyle.

Many Diseases, One Answer

A low-fat, low-protein diet is just as effective at avoiding cancer as it is for losing weight and preventing heart disease. There's no need to take special supplements or eat particular foods to treat individual ailments. As a matter of fact, that's counterproductive.

Dr. Campbell's 8 Principles of Food, Health, and Disease

Throughout his journey, Dr. Campbell came to some conclusions and put them together into eight principles that he believes represent what he's learned. He believes that these principles should be reflected in the way that we eat, the way that we treat our sick, the way we perceive the world, and the way that we think about health.

To reiterate, all that you have to do in order to avoid the vast majority of illnesses and debilitating conditions is to feed your body properly: eat a low-fat, low-protein, plant-based diet.

Principle 1: "Nutrition represents the combined activities of countless food substances. The whole is greater than the sum of its parts."

What Dr. Campbell means by this is that each food is made up of many different nutrients and chemicals that interact with each other to do things that none of the nutrients could do independently. The same theory applies in a grander scale to combining nutritious foods with each other.

The chemical reaction continues when the food enters your mouth and mixes with your saliva and digestive juices. Then the foods are carried into your bloodstream, causing certain reactions dictated by your body in an infinitely complex process that it has created as a means to fuel itself and fight disease efficiently.

His point is that touting the virtues of one specific food or nutrient is entirely too simplistic. Your body needs all of the different nutrients found in varied whole foods in order to create all of the reactions that it needs to thrive.

Principle 2: "Vitamin supplements are not a panacea for good health."

This principle carries forth the idea that you need a wide variety of nutrients in whole-food form in order to give your body what it needs. There's no need to supplement with individual nutrients if you're eating a wide array of plant-based foods. Supplements can't replace nutritious food, and the excesses of the Western diet can't be masked by popping one pill or even twelve.

Using supplements in place of nutritious foods is simply sacrificing your long-term health for short-term gains that you probably won't recognize anyway. Dr. Campbell doesn't claim that the nutrients aren't important, because they are; he simply advocates consuming them in the form of food versus pills.

Principle 3: "There are virtually no nutrients in animal-based foods that are not better provided by plants."

Per bite, plant-based eating provides more usable nutrition than animal-based diets do. They have exponentially more antioxidants, vitamins, and fiber. They also have much less (or no) cholesterol and saturated fats in the form of long-chain triglycerides, which are the heart-stoppers.

Plants also have slightly less protein, but the protein that they do have is easier to process and isn't accompanied by the bad fats. The one essential vitamin that plants don't provide is vitamin B12. Even though it's present in nutrient-rich soils, very few soils today actually have a good supply, and even if they do, the vegetables are so sanitized in the production process that vitamin B12 is virtually eliminated. As a result, you may need to take an occasional B12 supplement.

Principle 4: "Genes do not determine disease on their own. Genes function only by being activated, or expressed, and nutrition plays a critical role in determining which genes, good and bad, are expressed."

Every single disease has a genetic root. Quite simply, if you don't have the genes already in your DNA to develop the disease, you won't get it. This applies to cancer, diabetes, and every other condition possible to contract. That's why so much research money is spent trying to isolate genes that cause the disease. The issue here is that not all genes are expressed all the time. If they aren't, then they aren't biochemically active and don't have any effect on health.

The thing about these dormant genes is that they won't be expressed unless they have the proper stimulators or environment. For example, you're not going to develop heart disease if you don't eat the saturated fats that encourage it or skip the antioxidants that prevent it. The China Study highlighted this fact; people with extremely similar ethnic backgrounds had vastly different disease rates depending upon diet and lifestyle.

A final argument here is that disease rates have risen so fast over the last few decades that there's no way that genetics alone are responsible. There's simply no biological way that gene structure could have altered that drastically in just a couple of generations.

Principle 5: "Nutrition can substantially control the adverse effects of noxious chemicals."

Our environment is full of toxic chemicals. They're in the air that we breathe, the surfaces that we touch, and the food and water that we eat and drink. Two of those we can control by drinking clean filtered water and eating organic foods, though there's still no guarantee. We can't always control what's in the air or on the surfaces that we touch.

That's where good nutrition comes in. The antioxidants in fresh whole produce and the fiber in produce and grains work to keep our systems free of junk and free radicals that poison us slowly and cause disease.

There's a certain level of personal responsibility that goes along with this theory too. An example given in the book is the acrylamides found in potato chips. It makes them toxic, but even if you take out the acrylamide, you're still ingesting white potatoes fried in oil and coated in salt. Not exactly the healthiest thing.

To take this a step further, consider the toxins that you can't avoid. Plant-based, low-fat, low-protein eating can eliminate many of them from your body before they have a chance to harm you.

Principle 6: "The same nutrition that prevents disease in its early stages (before diagnosis) can also halt or reverse disease in its later stages (after diagnosis)."

Diseases such as cancer don't just pop up overnight. They take months and years to form. For example, cancer may begin growing in a woman's breast for a decade without being detected. That doesn't mean that there's nothing you can do about it though. Research is proving that cancer growth can be reversed, or cured if you will, even after the malignant cells are already present.

This doesn't apply to all diseases; for example, once your body develops an autoimmune disease, it's often unstoppable. Your body has literally turned upon itself. Still, the damage can be halted and sometimes be reversed with the proper lifestyle changes. The point here is that even if you're already sick, don't give up hope or turn away from modifying your eating habits, because you still stand a fighting chance.

Principle 7: "Nutrition that is truly beneficial for one chronic disease will support health across the board."

Any diet that targets a specific disease is more about good marketing than good science. Though diseases manifest in many different ways, their roots are similar; often they're caused by the same, or extremely similar, biochemical processes. Because of this, a healthful diet targeted at preventing heart disease is also going to protect you from cancer, strokes, and many other conditions that harm you.

Dr. Campbell's point here is exactly that: eat a low-fat, low-protein, plant-based diet to avoid any disease and to treat any condition with which you may be afflicted. What's good for the goose is good for the gander.

Principle 8: "Good nutrition creates health in all areas of our existence. All parts are interconnected."

Food isn't just something that you put into your body; it's fuel that affects all areas of your well-being. What you eat protects you from disease (or creates an environment in which it can thrive.), as we've already discussed. Food also provides fuel that your body uses for energy, digestion, and even mood regulation and self-esteem. What you eat affects how you look, how you feel, and how healthy you are.

That's not all, though. What you eat affects other areas of your life as well. It affects your energy levels, which affects your physical fitness, and it also affects the environment. A whole-food, plant-based diet has a much smaller carbon footprint than an animal-based diet does.

Why Are These Principles So Important?

Dr. Campbell's eight principles are important for a few different reasons. First and foremost, they help to reduce confusion about why a low-fat, low-protein, plant-based diet is so good for you. They also show that fad diets and the latest diet pills aren't the way to go if you're looking for long-term health. Finally, they show that it's easy to be healthy; you don't have to jump through hoops, pay a fortune for a diet plan, or waste time counting calories and restricting yourself.

As Dr. Campbell says, you can relax. Take a breath, step back from all of the hype that's going to be thrown at you every time you turn on the television, and just be healthy.

The China Study Results

The China Study showed that the closer a person is to a 100 percent plant-based diet low in fat and protein, the less his or her chances are of developing illnesses. Diseases of affluence are practically nonexistent with such a lifestyle; as a matter of fact, there were no causes of death by heart disease in some of the villages that ate only a plant-based diet. The same thing goes for cancer, stroke, obesity, and all of the other conditions that commonly affect those who eat a Western diet.

The most important result of the China Study is that we can avoid disease and live long, healthy lives just by giving up animal products in favor of whole, low-fat, low-protein, plant-based foods. It really is that simple.

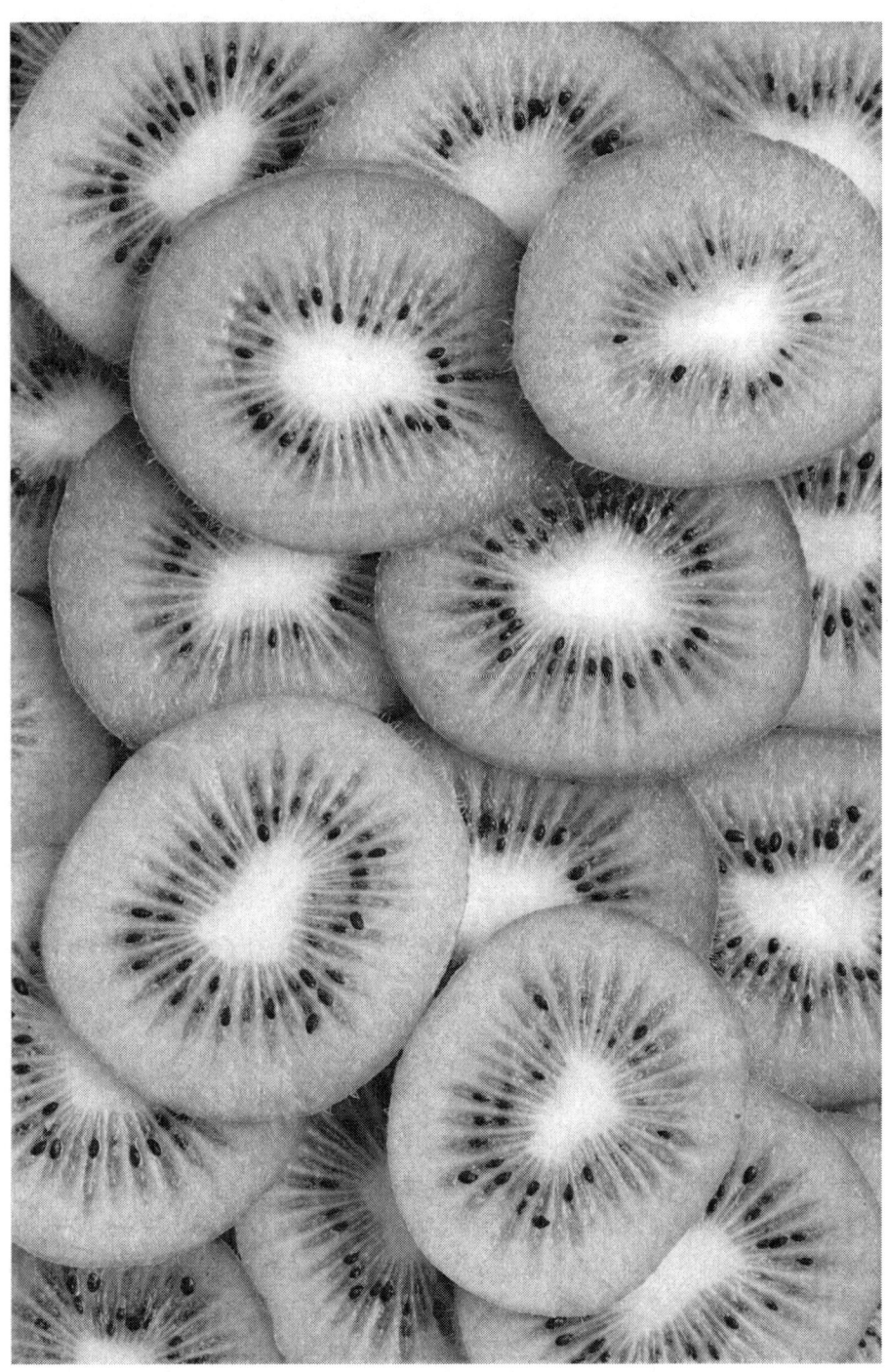

Kiwis make a delicious garnish for fruit dishes and are high in vitamin C.

3

BAD FOODS:
HOW YOUR DIET IS MAKING YOU SICK AND
MAKING YOU GAIN WEIGHT

You probably already have a general idea about how bad processed food and saturated animal fats are for you. Unfortunately though, you may only know about the superficial side effects: obesity, high cholesterol, heart disease, and the like. Those are bad enough, but they're only the tip of the American health crisis iceberg. We are quite literally eating ourselves to death, one cheeseburger at a time.

The bad part is that the powers that be really aren't getting the word out like they should, due mostly to politics and economics. As a matter of fact, a couple of decades ago, the agencies that monitor nutrition actually supported the nutritional value of fast food burgers.

Unless you've been living under the sea for the past decade, you've surely heard about and seen the health of America—and Western civilization in general—decline rapidly. All of the major diseases of affluence are escalating at an alarming rate, and there's no sign of an end to that trend. It's apparently a freight train that isn't going to stop until it hits the wall.

The most alarming result of this, perhaps, is that diseases such as type 2 diabetes, which has historically been found primarily in older adults, are now raging rampant in children. We're shortening our life spans and decreasing our quality of life in the name of gluttony and expedience; what's worse is we're teaching our kids these habits from a very young age and putting them at even higher risk.

Consider these facts for just a minute. According to the Center for Disease Control and Prevention (CDC):

- Every year, six hundred thousand Americans die from heart disease; that's one in four deaths.

- Type 2 diabetes has nearly tripled since 1980.

- More than one-third of American adults are clinically obese.

Our government is starting to wise up, though. The CDC recommends a diet low in sodium, fat, and cholesterol, and rich in fruits and vegetables in order to avoid heart disease. It's the number one killer in our country. What's troubling is that it's nearly 100 percent avoidable by switching to a low-fat, plant-based diet and eliminating processed foods.

Let's take a look at some of these diseases individually just to touch on some individual facts so that you can see exactly how quickly the Western diet is destroying our lives.

Heart Disease

As we've already discussed, heart disease is at an all-time high, and you probably won't be surprised to learn that the biggest risk factors for this deadly disease are other diseases of affluence: high blood pressure, high cholesterol, and obesity. Smoking is a huge contributor too. But what do all of these risks have in common? They're Western diseases. Specifically, they're American diseases, all causing the great American death—heart disease. And they're all avoidable by simply changing your lifestyle.

Risk factors aren't always causes, though. They're simply markers that accompany the disease; commonalities that our doctors use to identify whether or not someone is at risk of developing heart disease. In this instance, though, high cholesterol, one of the biggest risk factors, really is a cause.

Cholesterol is created by your body for a few different purposes; namely, it shuttles around fat-soluble vitamins from one place to another. Obviously, you need this cholesterol to function. The problem arises when you eat too many foods containing saturated fats in the form of long-chain triglycerides, because that's the source of bad cholesterol.

Why Animal-Sourced Saturated Fats Are Bad

The problem isn't necessarily the fact that your body is making cholesterol; it's the type of cholesterol that you need to worry about. There are two kinds: LDL, which is the "bad" cholesterol that clogs your arteries, and HDL which is the "good" cholesterol that lowers your LDL levels. The reason that animal-sourced saturated fat is so bad for you is because it's composed of long-chain triglycerides, or LCTs.

These LCTs are processed in your liver and turned into various fatty substances, including LDL cholesterol. If you eat too much, your liver just keeps making it, and it cycles through your bloodstream and can eventually end up sticking to the walls of your arteries and causing atherosclerosis—the beginning of cardiovascular disease.

Type 2 Diabetes

The typical American diet is packed with sugars, starches, and refined flours that have no fiber or even quality protein to slow the absorption of glucose down. Eating white breads, chips, and drinking sodas is essentially equivalent to dumping it straight into your bloodstream. We've already discussed what happens when you do this long-term, so it's really no wonder that type 2 diabetes is on the rise. Quite the opposite is more curious, actually: considering the way that we eat poorly and rarely exercise, it's a wonder that more people don't have it type 2 diabetes.

Obesity

Though all of the diseases of affluence are closely related, obesity is a common factor amongst them all. It's one of the "signal" diseases that indicate the probability of developing other diseases, and it's a sign of poor health in general.

Two out of three Americans are overweight, and one in three adults are clinically obese. Your body simply isn't designed to carry that much extra weight. It damages you inside and out. Your organs have to work harder, your joints are taxed with every step, and your muscles are under constant unnecessary strain.

Add to that the fact that strength training or cardiovascular workouts aren't typically at the top of an obese person's to-do list, and you've got the perfect recipe for an early death or a disease-ridden existence, thanks exclusively to poor dietary and lifestyle choices.

The recipes in Chapters 6–11 are naturally geared to help you lose weight by focusing on whole, plant-based dishes that are low in calories and high in fiber and good cholesterol. The China Study Diet wasn't conceived of as a weight-loss plan, but it achieves that goal by replacing high-fat and processed foods with healthful alternatives. In many ways, it's exactly the kind of diet that humans were genetically designed to eat.

Cancer

Believe it or not, this falls into the "diseases caused by diet" category as well. Most people are under the impression that cancer is genetic and random but, in the vast majority of cases, it isn't. As we've already discussed, even if you're genetically predisposed to cancer, its development is connected to having an environment that it can thrive in.

Free radicals, man-made trans fats, poor immunity, toxic chemicals, and many other factors brought about by a diet packed with saturated fats, empty carbohydrates, and hormones and preservatives used in animal products and processed foods contribute to activating cancer cells. If you eat a diet weighted heavily in that direction, the few fruits and vegetables that you consume simply can't eliminate the garbage fast enough to prevent it from damaging your body.

Peripheral Effects of a Poor Diet

Heart disease, obesity, diabetes, and other diseases are the worst conditions related to an animal-based diet and poor exercise habits, but they're certainly not the only ones. Being overweight and unhealthy has numerous side effects, including:

- Chronic fatigue
- Acne or splotchy skin
- Bad breath
- Poor teeth
- Indigestion
- Constipation

The list goes on. Animal protein is more difficult to digest than plant proteins, and your body processes animal fats differently too. We'll get into that in the next chapter, so let's move on.

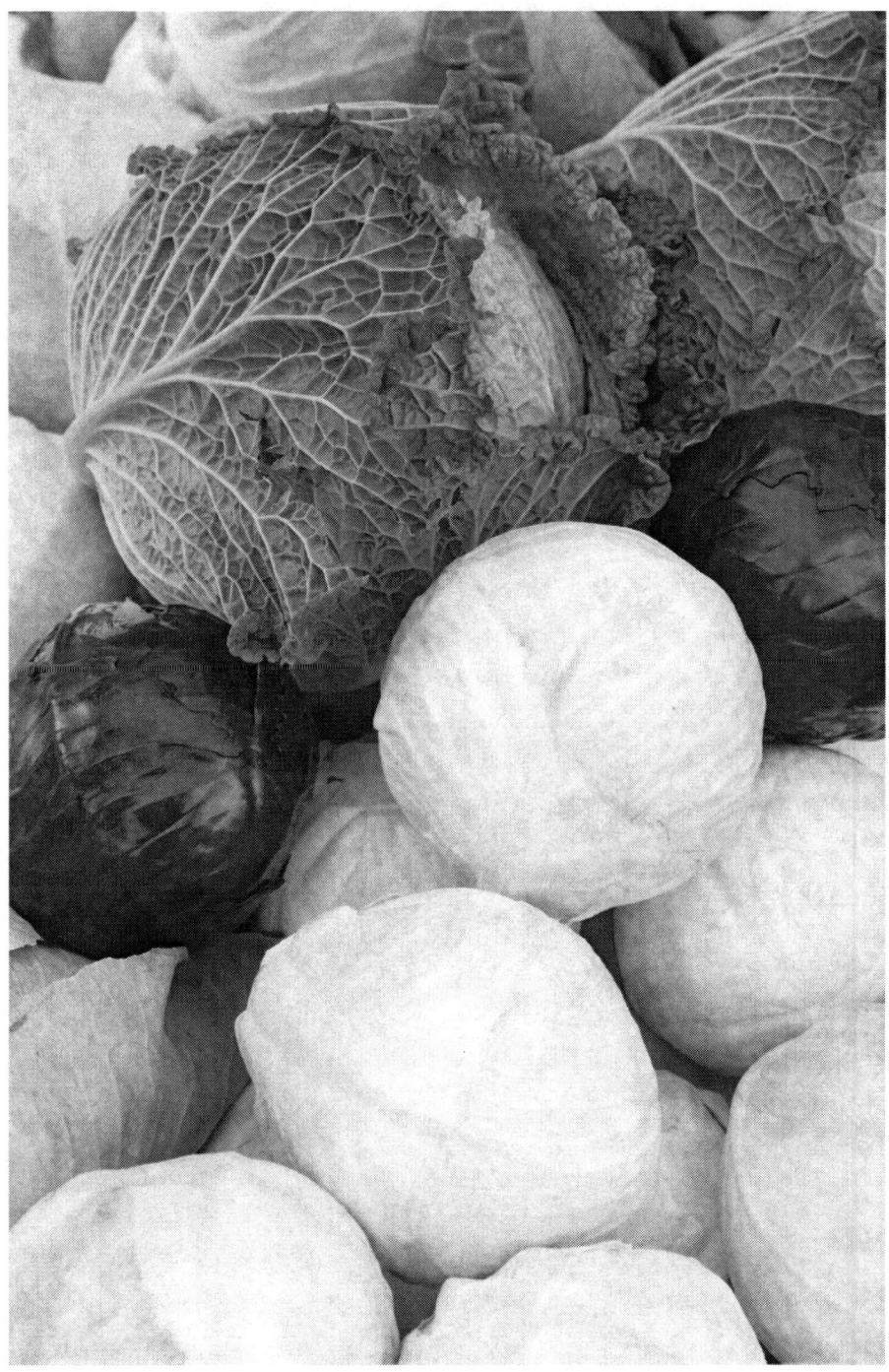

Around the world, cabbage is prepared in a variety of ways, including steamed, stewed, pickled, braised, sautéed, and raw.

4

GOOD FOOD: TRANSFORMING YOUR HEALTH WITH THE CHINA DIET

Just as you can kill yourself with food, you can also cure yourself. There are many documented cases of actual disease reversal seen in people who switched to a clean, plant-based diet rich in nutrients and low in fat and simple carbohydrates. Your body truly does have the ability to keep itself healthy and to heal itself if you just give it the proper tools. We're going to teach you how to do that, and explain why a plant-based diet can transform your health.

There are four basic components of nutrition that make a plant-based diet superior to an animal diet from a health perspective. Each area contributes greatly to your overall health, which is why there is no such thing as a diet specifically created to treat certain diseases; your body operates on a delicate balance, and each part must be in good working order for the whole body to be so.

Protein

Since protein seems to be the hang-up that most people have about switching to a plant-based diet, we'll start here. For eons, meat has been associated with both protein and affluence. If you consider that most of the Western diet shows that the more you have, the less healthfully you eat, you can imagine how well this is working out for us as a civilization. We're already programmed to view meat as a sign of success; modern-day nutrition now pushes us toward it as the only means of healthful protein. That's simply not the truth.

It's true that protein is vital to our survival. It makes up the fibers of our muscles as well as functions as enzymes, hormones, and structural transporters, just to name a few roles. Protein strands wear out and must be replaced regularly. The only way that you can do that is by eating foods that have proteins. The amino acids are ingested, then act as building blocks for your body to shape into whatever form of protein that your body needs.

What the China Study suggests, however, is that the concept of meat equaling protein and protein equaling meat is a fallacy. There are other suitable sources of protein, and those sources are plants.

Meeting Your Amino Acid Needs

This is, without a doubt, the biggest argument against using plants as the primary source of protein. There are fifteen to twenty different types of amino acids, depending upon how they're divided. Your body can make all but about eight of them. These eight are referred to as essential amino acids because we need them to thrive but must get them from food sources. It just so happens that all eight essential amino acids are present in animal proteins, primarily because their structure and ratios are so similar to ours. Milk and eggs are actually the closest match for us. Plants, on the other hand, do not have all of the essential amino acids available from any single source.

Before you automatically agree then that animal protein is obviously the best "quality" protein source, you may be interested to know that the most complete, perfect protein source for humans is . . . other humans. Obviously that's not an option, but it does throw a bit of weight against the entire, "we're obviously meant to eat meat because it's a complete protein" argument.

How, then, do you meet your protein needs with plants? Easy — you eat a wide variety of plants, nuts, and legumes. By doing that, it's easy to get all of your amino acids. This is yet another reason why there is no specific group of foods that are great to treat specific conditions: you need to eat a variety of plants in order to get all that you need to stay healthy.

Protein and Cancer

The USDA recommended daily allowance for protein is around 55 grams, depending upon sex and age. That typically equates to 20 to 30 percent of your daily caloric intake. Dr. Campbell was intrigued by an obscure study in which the protein intake of rats was manipulated in order to observe liver cancer occurrences.

One group of rats was fed a 20 percent protein diet, and the other group was fed a 5 percent protein diet. Amongst the rats that were fed the higher protein, every single rat contracted liver cancer or its precursor lesions. In the group who had only 5 percent, not a single one of them got liver cancer or lesions.

These findings piqued his interested and actually started Dr. Campbell down the road of researching the link between cancer and protein consumption. This was, and still is, a major focus of his research, and he didn't just find correlations, he discovered actual causal relationships between protein consumption and some types of cancer.

Stopping Cancer in Its Tracks

Dr. Campbell designed his experiments in the area of protein and cancer carefully because he knew that it would be the subject of close scrutiny. As a matter of fact, he was a bit skeptical himself when he started. To completely oversimplify the process, he administered dosages of a carcinogen to ten different groups of rats, then he manipulated the amount of protein that they consumed.

Rats eating average amounts of dietary protein (20 percent) developed precancerous foci, while their counterparts who consumed lower amounts of protein did not.

To take the research a step further, Dr. Campbell tested again using different types of protein, including animal protein in the form of casein, wheat protein, and soy protein. Strangely enough, only the animal protein had any effect on the development of precancerous cells, even at the higher levels of carcinogen administration.

The final part of his study included switching the protein levels on some of the rats who had already developed full-blown tumors. The results with the casein rats were what you might think by now: the ones whose intake of protein was reduced had significantly less tumor growth than their high-protein-eating counterparts.

These findings are spectacular from a research point of view; if it were a chemical rather than animal protein that had been shown to have this direct effect on cancer growth, the news would have already been shouted from the rooftops. Instead, the word is being spread quietly, one reader at a time. But it is spreading!

Vitamins and Antioxidants

Vitamins and antioxidants are perhaps the most important benefits that a plant-based diet has to offer. You can easily obtain every single vitamin and mineral that your body needs with the exception of vitamin B6 from plants. Your body needs antioxidants to neutralize free radicals that, when left to roam free, wreak all kinds of havoc within your body.

Free radicals cause damage to your skin in the form of age spots and wrinkles, and they also cause skin cancer. They promote dull hair, heart disease, eye disease, and various forms of internal cancer as well. But what are free radicals, and why can they do so much harm?

Free radicals are cells that have become unstable due to a lost ion. This may occur because another free radical stole it, or it could just be the result of normal bodily functions, such as breathing. Your body makes a certain amount of free radicals to carry toxins out of your body, but exposure to chemicals and toxins via food, respiration, and your environment cause too many to be produced.

A loose free radical is dangerous because cells don't like to be unstable. In order to stabilize itself, a cell will steal ions from other cells, thereby creating more free radicals. Antioxidant vitamins neutralize these cells by attaching to the free radicals and carrying them out of your body, preventing further damage.

Some of these vitamins and antioxidants have regenerative powers too. They can reduce the appearance of wrinkles, and stop or even reverse deadly diseases such as cancer and heart disease. In short, you want to have as many of these little helpers in your diet as possible.

Eat the Rainbow!

The best way to ensure that you're getting all of the vitamins and antioxidants that you need is to eat produce in a variety of colors. Often the pigment of the fruit or vegetable is related to the vitamin they contain, so a wide range of colors deliver many different vitamins.

Eat a Variety of Greens for Good Health

Green leafy vegetables are great sources of just about every vita-
min and mineral, but you need to switch them up from time to
time because eating just one green vegetable, such as broccoli or
spinach, long-term in significant amounts can cause kidney stones
due to the oxalic acid levels. Yet another reason to mix things up!

Oxidative stress on your eyes can be alleviated by antioxidants, and they can even help lower blood cholesterol in order to keep your veins and heart healthy. Even if you're still sometimes eating meat, you need to eat plenty of fresh fruits and vegetables to be at your best!

Fiber Keeps You Clean and Disease-Free

Junk foods, animal proteins, and processed foods create a nasty buildup in your intestinal tract that causes everything from gas to cancer, but the fiber in fruits and vegetables acts like a broom and sweeps your intestines and the rest of your digestive tract clean.

The average person carries around about five pounds of fecal matter in their gut at any given time because of the backup caused by Western eating that just sits there, promoting illness and disease.

Another benefit of fiber is that it slows down digestion so that you're not getting a big blast of sugar into your bloodstream all at once. The sugars in fruits and vegetables have to be extracted from the fiber so the process is slow and steady instead of rapid such as it is when you eat refined foods. This helps to prevent sugar spikes but it also helps to prevent cravings, thus keeping you from reaching for that bag of candy bars.

Good Plant Fats

Your body needs fat for various uses. Primarily, there are vitamins that are fat-soluble, which means that your body can't absorb them without the presence of fat. These include vitamins A, D, E, and K, all of which are vital to your health and well-being. Cholesterol is actually one of the vehicles that your body creates to deliver these vitamins throughout the body. It's only when there is too much LDL (bad) cholesterol in your system that there's a problem.

Your body also uses fat as fuel when you're low on carbohydrates. You actually have an extremely intricate fuel system at work twenty-four hours per day. Your body chooses what source of fuel to use for what job. It prefers carbs but if you don't have any of those, it moves on to fats. If you don't have any fats, it moves on to protein, which is a bad thing—we've already discussed that your body needs that protein for important functions.

The difference between plant fats and animal fats, though, is significant. And trans fats warrant mention because they're absolutely lethal: They were created by humans in order to make oils more shelf-stable. However, your body doesn't know what to do with them. They float around and cause clogged arteries that lead to heart disease and stroke. Trans fats aren't present at all in plant fats.

Many store-bought oils, including olive oil, are still heavily processed and have lost many of the nutrients that they once contained. When you choose fats, choose healthful ones such as virgin coconut oil. It has numerous health benefits and is made mostly of short-chain triglycerides, which your body converts into short-chain fatty acids and burns mostly as fuel. Because it's broken down in the gut instead of in the liver with pancreatic fluid, your body treats coconut oil more like a carbohydrate than a fat, and thus it gets used up first.

A final advantage to using oils with medium-chain triglycerides is that although they do raise the level of LDL cholesterol in your blood, MCTs also raise the level of HDL (good) cholesterol. This is important because HDL controls the levels of LDL by carrying the excess out of your body. When it comes down to it, it's the ratio of LDL to HDL that really matters.

We've covered the main reasons that making the switch to a low-fat, low-protein, plant-based diet that's free from processed foods is the way to go if you want to be healthy, so now let's get in to the recipes. We're going to share some of our very best salads, soups, entrées, sides, and desserts with you, all designed according to the standards set forth in the China Study.

You're going to be surprised by just how easy and delicious it can be to eat foods that are fabulous for you.

PART 2

The China Study Diet Recipes

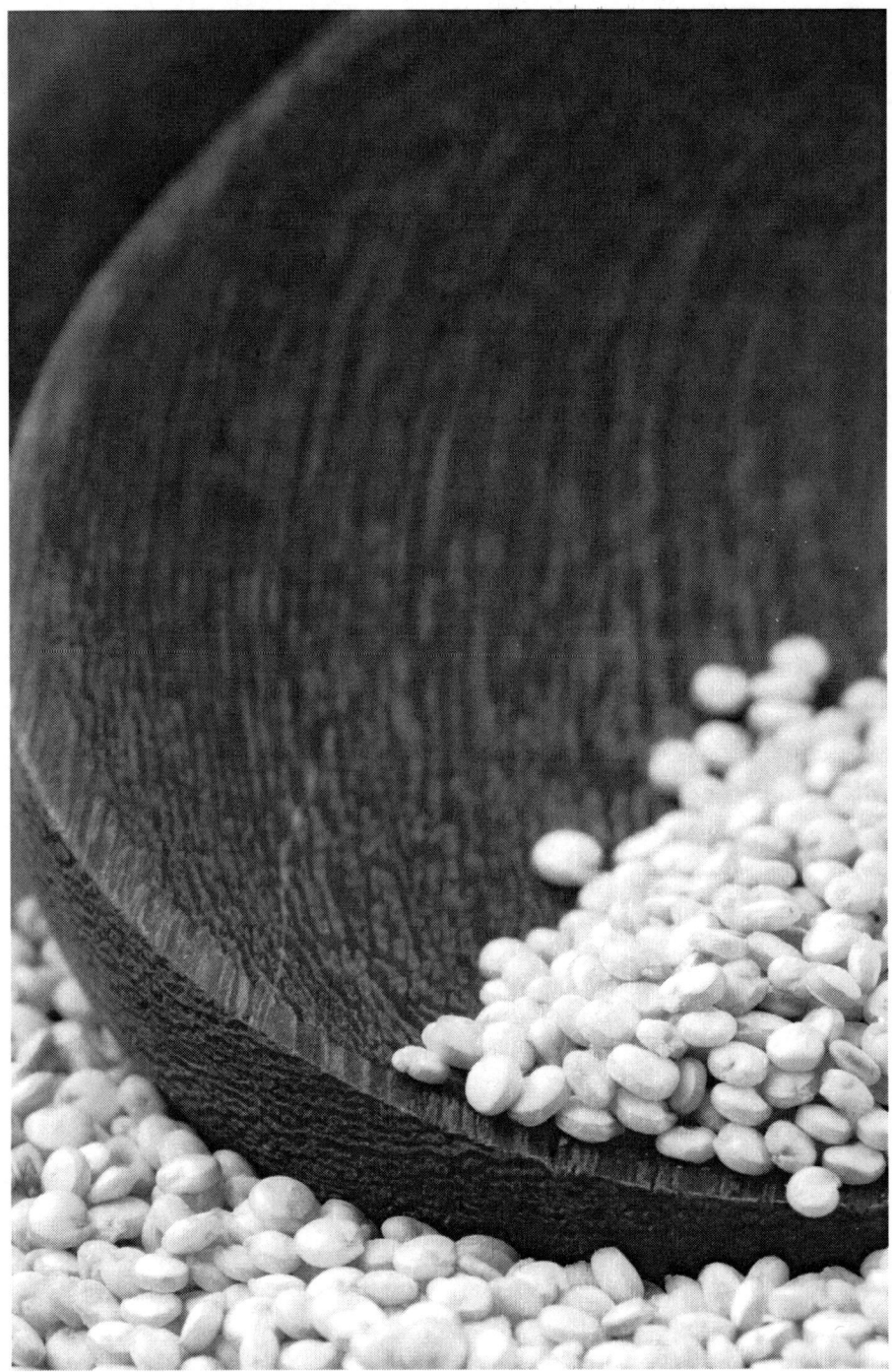

Quinoa is a great source of both protein and healthful fats, two nutrients that can be hard to get enough of on a strictly plant-based diet.

5

7-DAY MEAL PLAN FOR OPTIMUM HEALTH AND WEIGHT LOSS

The following is a week's worth of meal plans to help ease you into the China Study Diet. The snacks are foods allowed on the diet, and the breakfast, lunch, dinner, and dessert choices are recipes from Chapters 6–11. Feel free to follow these recommendations to the letter or create meal plans based on your preferences. By gradually replacing fatty, processed food in your diet and transforming your eating habits, weight loss will occur naturally in conjunction with a moderate exercise regimen. If you have any concerns about changing your diet or about starting an exercise plan, please consult your doctor.

DAY 1

Breakfast
Tropical Island Shake

Snack
Raw almonds, ¼ cup

Lunch
Tomato and Eggplant Salad

Dinner
Grilled Tofu Kabobs with Red Pepper Sauce
Savory Quinoa

Dessert
Bountiful Bread Pudding

DAY 2

Breakfast
Bright Day Citrus Smoothie

Snack
Cooked quinoa with cinnamon, ⅓ cup

Lunch
Chunky Vegetarian Chili

Dinner
Quinoa-Stuffed Butternut Squash
Oven-Roasted Vegetable Medley

Dessert
Bake-Less No Face Cookies

DAY 3

Breakfast
No Bake Fruity Nutty Bars

Snack
Blueberries, 1 cup

Lunch
Amazing Kale Soup

Dinner
Tofu Turkey Roast
Oven-Baked Potato Medley

Dessert
Berry Picnic Pie

DAY 4

Breakfast
Florida Key Lime Smoothie

Snack
Unsweetened applesauce, 1 cup

Lunch
Mexican Bean Salad

Dinner
Lentil and Vegetable Casserole
Brussels with a Kick

Dessert
Sweet Berry, No Dairy Parfait

DAY 5

Breakfast
Strawberry-Banana Smoothie

Snack
Celery with almond butter, ¼ cup

Lunch
Creamy Corn Chowder

Dinner
Moroccan Vegetable Curry
Sautéed Kale with Garlic

Dessert
Easy Peach Cobbler

DAY 6

Breakfast
Breakfast Granola Bars

Snack
Carrot sticks with hummus, ¼ cup

Lunch
Creamy Tomato Soup
Greek-Inspired Potato Salad

Dinner
Tempeh Fajita Filling
Spinach with Mushrooms and Peppers

Dessert
Coconut Cookies

DAY 7

Breakfast
Green Giant Smoothie

Snack
Mandarin orange, 1

Lunch
Chinese Hot and Sour Soup
Spinach and Orange Salad

Dinner
Flavorful Black Bean Burgers
Glazed Carrots

Dessert
Banana-Blueberry Sorbet

6

CHINA STUDY DIET BREAKFASTS

Summer Berries Breakfast Smoothie

Frozen berries work just as well as fresh berries in this recipe. Be sure that they have not been sweetened with added sugar. This breakfast smoothie is loaded with antioxidants and vitamin C.

- 1½ cups berries (any combination of blueberries, blackberries, and raspberries)
- 2 cups plain almond milk
- 1 teaspoon pure vanilla extract
- 1 teaspoon raw honey
- Handful of ice cubes

1. Put the berries in a blender and blend on high until smooth.

2. Add the almond milk, vanilla, honey, and ice cubes, and blend on high until thick and creamy.

3. Serve immediately.

Makes 2 large or 4 small smoothies.

Green Giant Smoothie

Kale is one of the most nutritious of the dark leafy greens, but it can be a little bitter in its raw form. The use of orange juice and pears in this smoothie adds just the right touch of acidity and sweetness to satisfy.

- 1 cup fresh orange juice
- 1 cup chopped kale
- 1 cup chopped spinach
- 2 fresh pears, cored and chopped
- Handful of ice cubes

1. Combine the orange juice, kale, spinach, and pears in a blender, and blend on high until smooth.

2. Add the ice cubes and blend on high until thick and creamy.

3. Serve immediately.

Makes 2 large or 4 small smoothies.

Florida Key Lime Smoothie

If you like the taste of key lime pie, you'll love this smoothie. Loaded with vitamin C, a good amount of protein, and healthy fats, it's a wholesome drink that tastes like dessert.

- 2 cups unsweetened coconut milk
- ¼ cup key lime juice
- ¼ cup raw honey
- 2 scoops egg white powder
- 1 teaspoon ground flaxseed

1. Combine all the ingredients in a blender and blend until smooth.

2. Serve immediately.

Makes 2 large or 4 small smoothies.

Strawberry-Banana Smoothie

This smoothie is a breakfast favorite for kids and those who like something sweet to start the day, but it's also healthy and filling. You can freeze servings in individual airtight containers for about 2 hours and it becomes a frozen treat.

- 1 pint strawberries, stemmed
- 2 large bananas, sliced
- 1 teaspoon honey
- 1 teaspoon pure vanilla extract
- 3 cups unsweetened coconut milk or plain almond milk
- Handful of ice cubes

1. Combine the strawberries, bananas, honey, and vanilla in a blender, and blend on high until smooth.

2. Turn the blender on low and gradually pour in the milk until it is fully incorporated.

3. Add the ice cubes, turn blender on high, and blend until thick and creamy. Serve immediately or freeze.

Makes 2 large or 4 small smoothies.

Tropical Island Shake

When you want something that makes you feel like you're basking on a beach, this will do the trick. Similar to a piña colada, this shake is full of the flavors of summer.

- 1 cup cream of coconut
- 1 cup unsweetened canned pineapple
- ½ cup canned pineapple juice
- 1 teaspoon lime juice
- Handful of ice cubes

1. Combine the cream of coconut, pineapple, pineapple juice, and lime juice in a blender, and blend on high until smooth.

2. Turn the blender on low and blend until it is fully incorporated.

3. Add the ice cubes and blend on high until thick and creamy. Serve immediately.

Makes 2 large or 4 small smoothies.

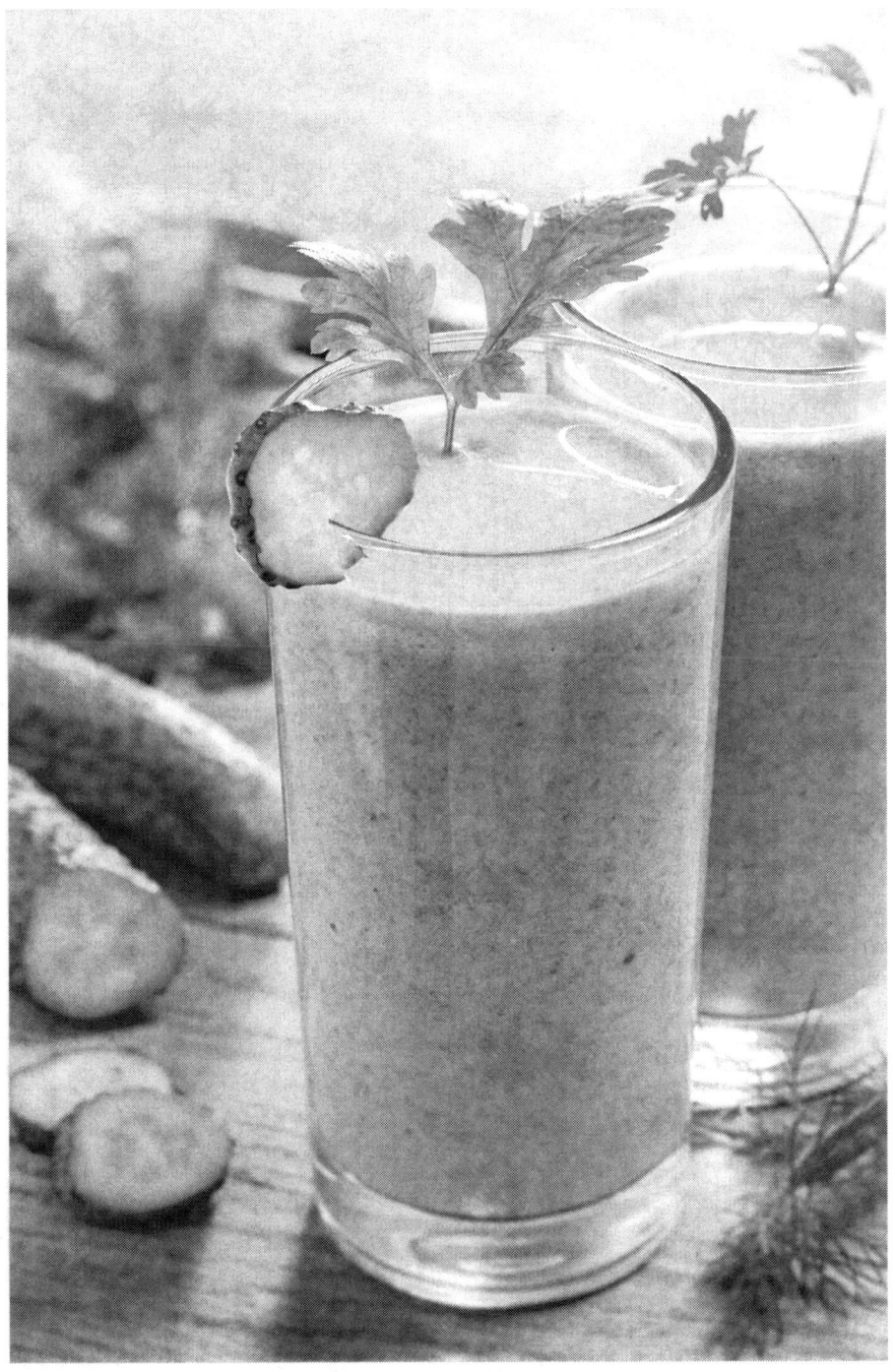

Freshly made juices and smoothies are a quick and easy way to get your recommended daily serving of fruits and vegetables.

Bright Day Citrus Smoothie

The flavors of this sweet and tangy smoothie are similar to the classic orange sherbet-vanilla ice-cream treat, but this drink is far better for you. It will separate if it sits for too long, so be sure to drink it right away.

- 2 cups unsweetened coconut milk or plain almond milk
- ¼ cup unsweetened frozen orange juice concentrate
- ½ cup canned pineapple juice
- 1 banana, sliced
- 1 teaspoon pure vanilla extract
- Handful of ice cubes

1. Combine the milk, orange juice concentrate, pineapple juice, banana, and vanilla in a blender, and blend on high until smooth.

2. Add the ice cubes and blend on high until thick and creamy. Serve immediately.

Makes 2 large or 4 small smoothies.

Breakfast Granola Bars

This recipe is far better for you than any commercial granola bars, which are often laden with high-fructose corn syrup and unhealthy grains. They bake quickly and will keep in an airtight container for up to 1 week.

- 1 teaspoon coconut oil
- 1 cup pecan pieces
- 1 cup pumpkin seeds
- 1 cup chopped walnuts
- 1 cup dried cranberries
- 1 cup dried apricots, chopped
- 1 cup unsweetened coconut flakes
- ¼ cup coconut oil, melted
- ½ cup almond butter
- ½ cup honey
- ¼ teaspoon pure vanilla extract
- ½ teaspoon salt
- 1 teaspoon ground cinnamon

1. Preheat the oven to 325 degrees F. Grease a 9 x 13 inch baking pan with the coconut oil and set aside.

2. In a large bowl, combine the pecans, pumpkin seeds, walnuts, cranberries, apricots, coconut flakes, and toss to mix well.

3. In a small saucepan over low heat, combine the melted coconut oil, almond butter, honey, vanilla, salt, and cinnamon, and heat just until the honey is completely melted.

4. Transfer the nut mixture to the baking pan, pressing down to spread it evenly. Pour the oil-honey mixture evenly over the top.

5. Bake for 35 to 40 minutes, or until golden. Let cool to room temperature before cutting into bars. Store in an airtight container for up to 1 week.

Makes 1 dozen bars.

Sweet Potato Breakfast Squares

These bars are moist and flavorful, and they come with all the fiber and beta-carotene that sweet potatoes provide. They don't freeze well but will keep for 1 week in an airtight container.

- ½ teaspoon coconut oil
- 2 large baked sweet potatoes
- 3 tablespoons almond flour
- 1 cup unsweetened coconut flakes
- ¼ teaspoon baking soda
- ¼ teaspoon cream of tartar
- ½ teaspoon ground cinnamon
- ¼ teaspoon salt
- ¼ teaspoon ground nutmeg
- 1 cup unsweetened golden raisins
- ¼ cup coconut oil, melted
- ½ cup honey

1. Preheat the oven to 350 degrees F. Grease a 9 x 13 inch baking pan with the coconut oil and set aside.

2. Split open the sweet potatoes and spoon the flesh into a large mixing bowl. Use a fork or hand mixer to mash the potatoes until smooth.

3. Stir in the almond flour, coconut flakes, baking soda, and cream of tartar until well combined, then add the cinnamon, salt, and nutmeg, and mix well. Add the raisins, melted coconut oil, and honey, stirring to incorporate.

4. Transfer the batter to the baking pan and smooth it into an even layre. Bake for 35 to 40 minutes or until a toothpick inserted into the center comes out clean.

5. Let cool for 1 hour before cutting into bars.

Makes 1 dozen bars.

No-Bake Fruity Nutty Bars

There are few snacks as beloved as chewy snack bars, and these make the perfect on-the-go breakfast. These bars hit all the right notes, with a combination of nuts, coconut, honey, and dried fruit. As a bonus, you don't even have to bake to enjoy these treats! The bars keep well, so make several batches at once.

- 2 cups raw pecan halves or pieces
- 2 cups raw walnut halves or pieces
- ½ teaspoon sea salt
- ½ teaspoon cinnamon
- ¼ teaspoon nutmeg
- 3 tablespoons plus ½ teaspoon coconut oil, melted

- ½ cup unsweetened shredded coconut
- ½ cup dried, unsweetened cranberries, chopped
- ½ cup dried, unsweetened cherries, chopped
- ½ cup raw honey

1. In a food processor or blender, grind the pecans and walnuts together until they are similar to breadcrumbs in consistency. Work in batches and be careful not to grind them too long or you will end up with pecan-walnut butter!

2. Pour the ground nuts into a large mixing bowl and add salt, cinnamon, and nutmeg, mixing well with your hands or a large spoon. Pour 3 tablespoons coconut oil over the mixture and blend well.

3. Stir in the shredded coconut, cranberries, and cherries until well mixed, then add the honey. Line a 9 x 13 inch baking pan with aluminum foil and lightly grease the bottom and sides with ½ teaspoon coconut oil. Use a spoon or sturdy spatula to spread the mixture evenly into the baking pan, pressing it down firmly.

4. Cover with foil and let sit for 3–4 hours before cutting into bars.

Makes 1 dozen bars.

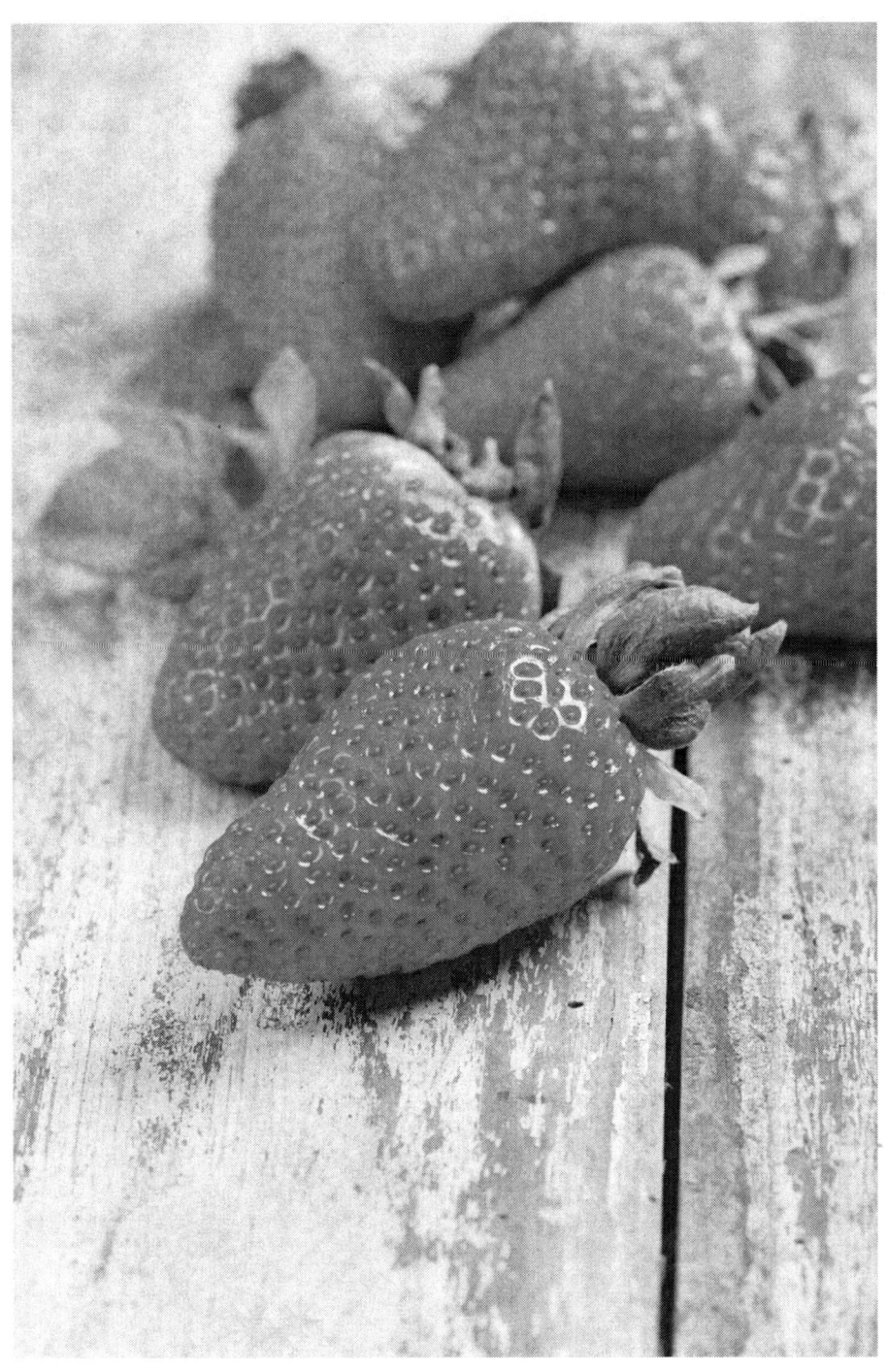

Strawberries are a great source of vitamin C and antioxidants.

7

CHINA STUDY DIET SALADS

Strawberry Walnut Salad

Strawberries are a great source of vitamin C and other antioxidants. Walnuts are an excellent source of omega-3 fatty acids, which are good for both heart health and cognitive function. These ingredients, combined with plenty of romaine lettuce, make this salad an especially healthful one. It's best dressed lightly with a simple vinaigrette.

- 2 cups torn romaine lettuce
- ½ cup halved cherry tomatoes
- ¼ cup diced red onion
- ¼ cup walnut halves
- ¼ cup balsamic vinaigrette of your choice
- ½ cup sliced fresh strawberries

---

1. In a large bowl, combine the lettuce, tomatoes, onion, walnuts, and vinaigrette. Toss well.

2. Gently fold in the strawberries and serve immediately.

Serves 2.

Warm Lentil and Bell Pepper Salad

Lentils are an excellent way to get a good dose of both iron and fiber into your meal. Cooked lentils will keep very well in the fridge for about 3 days, so make a large batch of them to toss into salads like this one or to add to soups and stews. You can use any type of lentil for this recipe.

- 2 tablespoons plus 1 teaspoon coconut oil, divided
- 2 cloves garlic, chopped
- 1 cup chopped Swiss chard
- ½ red bell pepper, chopped
- ½ yellow bell pepper, chopped
- ½ cup sliced fresh mushrooms
- ½ teaspoon salt
- ½ teaspoon paprika
- ¼ teaspoon freshly ground black pepper
- 1 cup cooked lentils
- 1 tablespoon balsamic vinegar
- 2 scallions, sliced

1. In a large heavy skillet, heat the 1 teaspoon of coconut oil over medium heat.

2. Once the oil is hot, add the garlic and sauté for 2 minutes. Add the Swiss chard, bell peppers, mushrooms, salt, paprika, and black pepper to the skillet, and sauté for about 3 minutes, or just until the peppers are slightly tender. Stir in the lentils, reduce the heat to low, and let simmer for 2 minutes.

3. Meanwhile, in a small bowl, whisk together the remaining 2 tablespoons of coconut oil and the balsamic vinegar, blending just until opaque.

4. To serve, spoon the salad onto plates, drizzle with the vinaigrette, and top with the scallions.

Serves 2.

Quinoa and Black Bean Salad

Quinoa is one of the best protein sources you can find among plant-based foods. It's actually a seed, but it's a wonderful stand-in for almost any grain food, including pasta. Quinoa is also a rich source of omega-3 fatty acids. Rinse and drain the quinoa at least twice before using, as you would for dried beans.

- ½ cup uncooked quinoa
- 1 teaspoon coconut oil
- 1 (15-ounce) can black beans, rinsed and well drained
- 2 cups diced fresh tomatoes
- 1 cup diced yellow bell pepper
- 2 tablespoons chopped scallions
- 2 teaspoons chopped jalapeño peppers
- 1 tablespoon chopped fresh cilantro
- 1 teaspoon chopped fresh basil
- ¼ teaspoon ground cumin
- ¼ teaspoon ground coriander
- 1 teaspoon salt
- ½ teaspoon freshly ground black pepper
- 4 teaspoons freshly squeezed lemon juice
- 2 cups chopped romaine lettuce

1. Cook the quinoa according to the package directions and drain any remaining water. Set aside to cool slightly.

2. In a medium skillet, heat the coconut oil over low heat. Add the beans, tomatoes, bell pepper, scallions, jalapeños, cilantro, basil, cumin, and coriander, and cook for 5 minutes.

3. Add the quinoa, season with the salt and pepper, and stir just until warmed through. Remove from the heat and sprinkle with the lemon juice.

4. To serve, divide the lettuce between two plates (or four if serving as an appetizer) and spoon the warm quinoa mixture on top.

Serves 2–4.

Vegan Mock Chicken Salad

Tempeh is one of the most versatile of the soy products to use as a substitute for more traditional animal-based ingredients. In this case, it stands in beautifully for chicken breast in a salad that is great over lettuce, in a wrap, or stuffed into avocado halves. Vegan mayonnaise is available in the natural foods or organic section of most supermarkets.

- 1 cup cubed tempeh
- ½ cup vegan mayonnaise
- 2 teaspoons Dijon mustard
- 2 teaspoons soy sauce
- 1 stalk celery, thinly sliced
- ¼ cup chopped sweet or bread-and-butter pickles
- ¼ cup chopped red onion
- 2 tablespoons chopped fresh parsley

1. Steam the tempeh for 10 minutes over boiling water (do not microwave); then transfer to a plate or cutting board to cool.

2. In a medium bowl, combine the mayonnaise, mustard, and soy sauce, stirring briskly with a fork until well blended.

3. Add the tempeh, celery, pickles, onion, and parsley to the bowl, and stir until well combined.

4. Cover and chill for at least 1 hour before serving.

Serves 2–4.

Smooth and Creamy Southwestern Dressing

This better-for-you version of a popular fast-food salad dressing is simple to make and wonderfully flavorful. It has just enough kick to please those who like it spicy, but not too much for everyone else. This will keep well in an airtight container for up to a week, although it may separate. If so, just stir briskly with a fork before using.

- 1 cup vegan mayonnaise
- 2 tablespoons water
- 1 tablespoon honey
- 2 teaspoons apple cider vinegar
- 2 teaspoons freshly squeezed lime juice
- 2 teaspoons chili powder
- 1 teaspoon garlic powder
- 1 teaspoon onion powder
- 1 teaspoon ground cumin
- Pinch of cayenne pepper

1. In a blender, combine the mayonnaise, water, honey, vinegar, and lime juice, and blend on low speed until smooth.

2. Add the chili powder, garlic powder, onion powder, cumin, and cayenne, and blend again until creamy and smooth.

3. Pour the dressing into an airtight container, and chill for at least 2 hours before serving.

Makes about 1 cup.

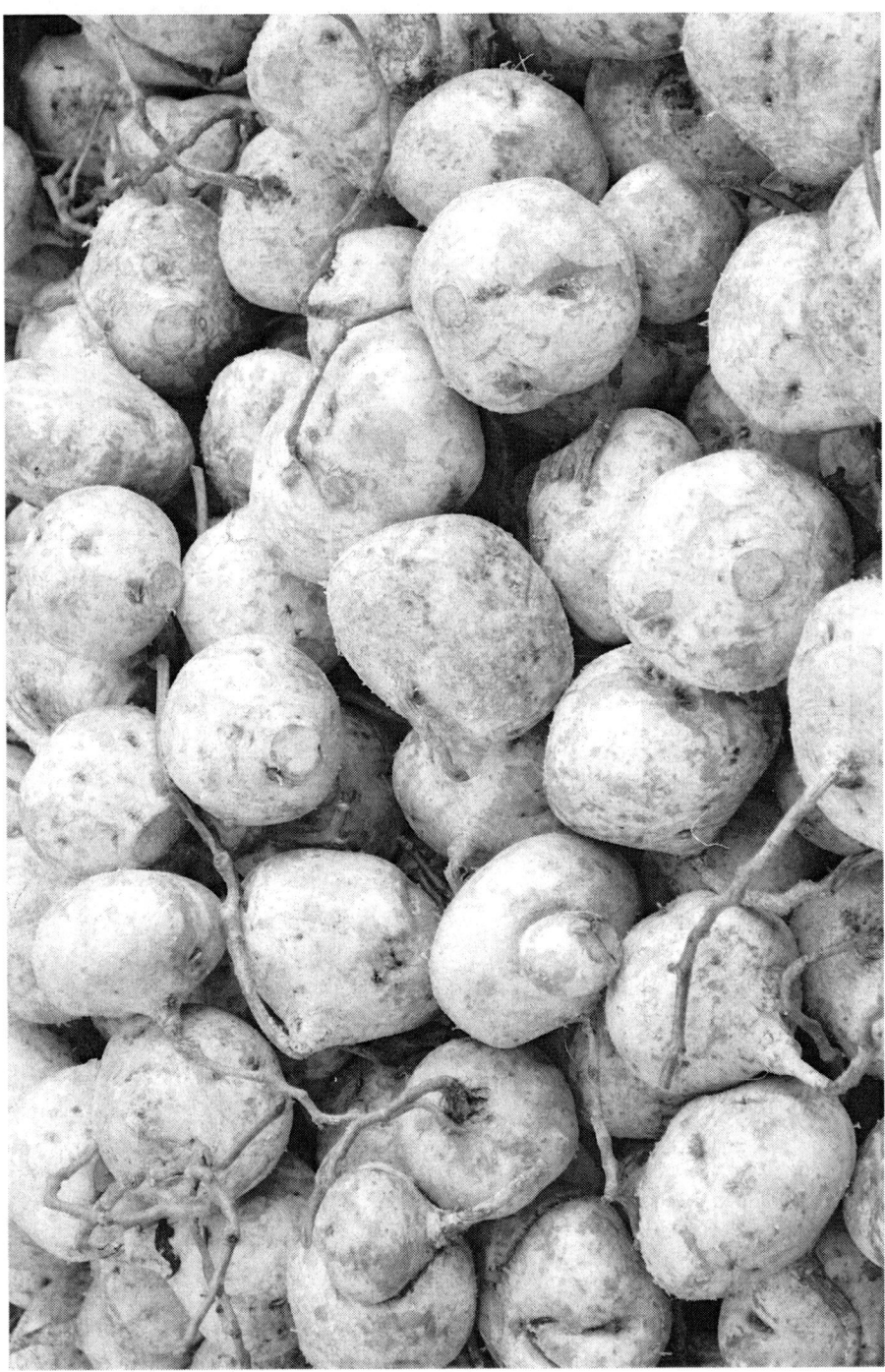

Jicama has a taste and texture similar to green apple, and makes a beautifully refreshing and crisp salad or slaw.

Thai-Style Jicama and Orange Slaw

Jicama has a taste and texture similar to green apple, and makes a beautifully refreshing, crisp salad or slaw. This recipe has just the right balance of spicy and sweet, which you can adjust to your individual taste with more or less heat. This slaw tastes even better the day after it's made.

- 1 large jicama, peeled and cut into thin strips
- 2 medium navel oranges, cut into chunks
- 1 large red bell pepper, chopped
- ½ small orange bell pepper, thinly sliced
- 1 small cucumber, diced
- 4 radishes, diced
- 3 sweet banana peppers, thinly sliced
- 3 Thai chili peppers, chopped
- ½ jalapeño pepper, chopped
- ½ cup chopped fresh cilantro
- Juice of 1 lime
- ½ teaspoon salt
- ¼ teaspoon freshly ground black pepper

1. In a medium bowl, combine the first 10 ingredients (through cilantro), and stir until well blended.

2. Stir in the lime juice, add the salt and pepper, and stir again until well blended.

3. Cover and chill for at least 1 hour before serving.

Serves 2.

Mexican Bean Salad

This delicious salad dresses up canned beans with fresh herbs and a lot of flavor. It's a great way to incorporate more iron, protein, and fiber-rich legumes into your diet. Feel free to play around with other bean varieties. For best results, make this a day ahead of serving.

- 1 (15-ounce) can black beans, rinsed and drained
- 1 (15-ounce) can kidney beans, rinsed and drained
- 1 (15-ounce) can great northern beans, rinsed and drained
- 1 green bell pepper, chopped
- 1 red bell pepper, chopped
- 1½ cups canned or frozen whole kernel corn (thawed), drained
- 1 medium red onion, chopped
- ½ cup coconut oil
- ½ cup red wine vinegar
- ¼ cup chopped fresh cilantro
- 2 tablespoons honey
- 2 tablespoons freshly squeezed lime juice
- 1 tablespoon freshly squeezed lemon juice
- 1 clove garlic, crushed
- 1 teaspoon salt
- ½ teaspoon freshly ground black pepper
- ½ teaspoon ground cumin
- ½ teaspoon chili powder
- Dash of red pepper sauce

1. In a medium bowl, combine the beans, bell peppers, corn, and onion, and stir until well blended.

2. In a separate bowl, whisk together the coconut oil, vinegar, cilantro, honey, lime and lemon juices, garlic, salt, pepper, cumin, and chili powder until smooth. Add the red pepper sauce to taste.

3. Pour the dressing over the vegetables and stir well. Cover and refrigerate for at least 2 hours.

Serves 8.

Spinach and Orange Salad

This simple but delicious salad is loaded with fiber, vitamin C, and iron. You can make the preparation even easier by using precut and prewashed baby spinach leaves. This is also wonderful with tangerines or fresh summer peaches.

- 2 large oranges
- 2 cups fresh spinach leaves, washed and dried
- ½ cup sliced fresh mushrooms
- ¼ cup sliced red onion
- ¼ cup pecan or walnut halves
- ¼ cup coconut oil
- ¼ cup red wine vinegar
- ¼ teaspoon salt
- ¼ teaspoon freshly ground black pepper

1. Remove the center membrane from the oranges, leaving the sections whole. Place into a medium bowl. Add the spinach, mushrooms, onion, and pecans and toss gently to combine.

2. In a small bowl, whisk together the coconut oil, vinegar, salt, and pepper until smooth.

3. Pour the dressing over the salad, and toss well to combine. Serve immediately.

Serves 2.

Mediterranean Cherry Tomato Salad

This salad is a variation on a dish popular in Italy and Southern France. It's traditionally served with fresh mozzarella but doesn't lack a thing without it. It's delicious on its own or in a wrap or sandwich. The salad will keep well in the fridge for up to 3 days and is a great lunch dish to take to work or school.

- 2 pints cherry tomatoes, halved
- 1 cup sliced green olives
- 1 (6-ounce) can sliced black olives, drained
- 2 scallions, chopped
- ⅓ cup pine nuts
- ½ cup coconut oil
- 2 tablespoons red wine vinegar
- 1 tablespoon honey
- 1 teaspoon dried oregano
- ½ teaspoon salt
- ¼ teaspoon freshly ground black pepper

1. In a large bowl, combine the tomatoes, olives, and scallions, tossing until well blended.

2. In a small dry skillet, toast the pine nuts over medium-low heat just until they are fragrant and slightly golden. Stir into the tomato mixture.

3. In a small bowl, whisk together the coconut oil, vinegar, honey, and oregano. Add the salt and pepper, and stir.

4. Gently stir the dressing into the salad. Cover and refrigerate for 1 hour before serving.

Serves 4.

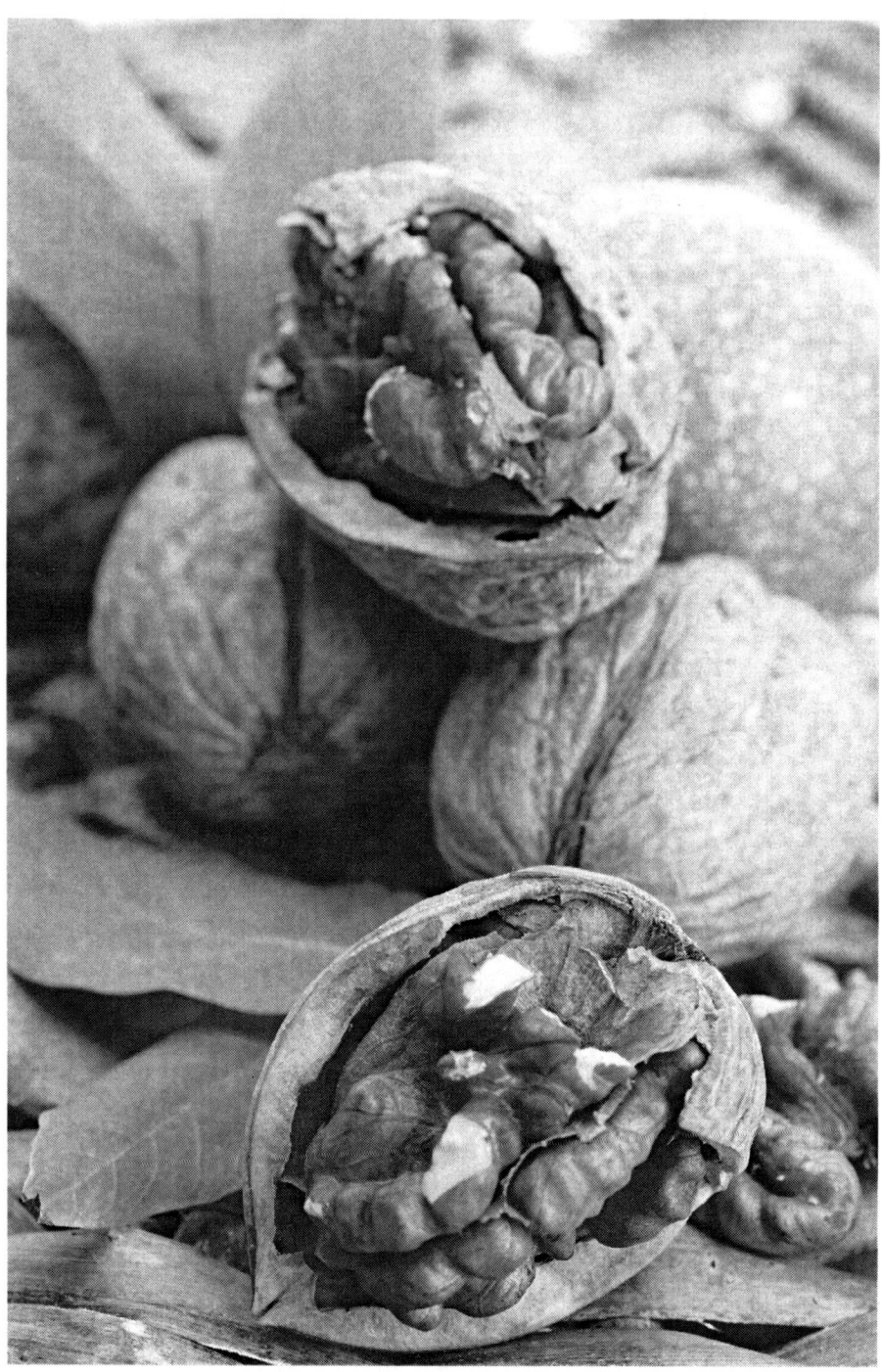

Walnuts are an excellent source of omega-3 fatty acids, which are good for both heart health and cognitive function.

Lime and Sweet Onion Dressing

This dressing is absolutely delectable and completely addicting. It's equally good on fresh fruit salads or over mixed greens, and it also makes a great dipping sauce for both fruits and vegetables. The dressing will keep well in an airtight container in the fridge for up to 3 weeks.

- 1 large sweet onion, peeled and quartered
- 1 clove garlic
- ¾ cup apple cider vinegar
- ¼ cup lime juice
- ¼ cup honey
- 1 teaspoon dry mustard
- 1 teaspoon salt
- 1½ cups coconut oil

1. In a blender, combine the onion, garlic, vinegar, lime juice, honey, dry mustard, and salt. Put the lid on the blender without the fill cap insert (hole should be open). Cover the hole loosely with a clean towel, and blend on low speed for 30 seconds.

2. With the blender still on low speed, remove the towel and very slowly pour the coconut oil into the blender. Blend until it's fully incorporated and the dressing is smooth and creamy.

Makes about 3 cups.

Marinated Mixed-Vegetable Salad

This salad is great as both a main dish and a side salad. The celery seed dressing lends a slightly unexpected flavor, similar to coleslaw. This is best prepared a day or two ahead to allow the flavors to intensify, but if you need to make it the day you're serving, marinate it for at least 3 hours.

For the dressing:
- 1 cup distilled white vinegar
- ¾ cup honey
- ¼ cup coconut oil
- 1 teaspoon celery seed
- 1 teaspoon salt
- ¼ teaspoon freshly ground black pepper

For the salad:
- 2 cups cucumber, peeled and thinly sliced
- 1 medium onion, thinly sliced
- 1 large yellow bell pepper, thinly sliced
- 2 cups thinly sliced carrots
- ½ cup chopped celery

Make the dressing:
1. In a small saucepan, combine the vinegar, honey, coconut oil, celery seed, salt, and pepper. Heat over medium heat, stirring occasionally, just until the honey is melted. Remove the pan from the heat, and allow the dressing to cool until just warm.

Make the salad:
1. In a large bowl, combine the cucumber, onion, bell pepper, carrots, and celery.

2. Pour the dressing over the vegetables and stir well to coat. Refrigerate overnight or for at least 3 hours.

Serves 4.

Grilled Fruit Salad

Grilling fruits caramelizes their natural sugars and brings out an extra layer of flavor. This salad is a great one for using summer fruits at their peak of ripeness. The recipe calls for grilling indoors, but it's excellent on the outdoor barbecue as well.

- 2 tablespoons coconut oil
- ½ teaspoon salt
- ¼ teaspoon freshly ground black pepper
- ¼ teaspoon chili powder
- 1 whole pineapple, cut into 1-inch chunks
- 1 medium cantaloupe, peeled and cut into 1-inch chunks
- 1 pint strawberries, hulled and halved
- 1 pound grapes

1. Heat a large stove-top grill over high heat.

2. Meanwhile, mix together the coconut oil, salt, pepper, and chili powder in a large bowl.

3. Arrange a single layer of pineapple and cantaloupe chunks on the grill, and use a pastry brush to brush with the oil mixture. Grill the fruit for 2 minutes, and then turn. Brush the cooked side with the oil mixture, and grill for 1 more minute. Transfer the cooked fruit to a large plate and set aside. Repeat until all of the pineapple and melon are cooked.

4. Toss the strawberries in the remaining oil mixture, and then transfer to the grill. Grill the strawberries for 1 minute and return to the large bowl. Add the pineapple, cantaloupe, and grapes, and stir to combine. Serve immediately.

Serves 4–6.

Greek-Inspired Potato Salad

Prepare this salad in advance for the perfect summer picnic salad or simply to make your workweek lunches something to look forward to. If you serve this flavorful dish at your next get-together, expect plenty of requests for this recipe.

- 12 small red potatoes (about 2 pounds)
- 2 quarts cold water
- 1 teaspoon salt
- ¼ cup chopped scallions
- ¼ cup coconut oil
- ¼ cup red wine vinegar
- 1½ teaspoons freshly squeezed lemon juice
- 1 teaspoon fresh lemon zest
- ½ teaspoon honey
- ½ teaspoon garlic powder
- ½ teaspoon onion powder
- ½ teaspoon sea salt
- ½ teaspoon freshly ground black pepper
- ¼ teaspoon dried oregano
- ¼ teaspoon dried rosemary, crushed
- Pinch of crushed red pepper flakes

1. In a large pot, cover the red potatoes with the cold water, and season with salt. Bring to a boil over high heat. Reduce the heat to medium and simmer for 20 minutes, or until the potatoes are tender. Drain and allow to cool to room temperature before refrigerating for 1 hour.

2. Slice the chilled potatoes and place in a large bowl. Add the scallions and mix well.

3. In a small bowl, whisk together the coconut oil, vinegar, lemon juice and zest, honey, garlic powder, onion powder, sea salt, black pepper, oregano, rosemary, and red pepper flakes.

4. Pour the dressing over the potatoes and toss well. Serve cold or at room temperature.

Serves 6.

Tomato and Eggplant Salad

Tomatoes and eggplants are both nightshades, and they work beautifully together, especially in this savory salad. This is an especially good dish to make late in summer when both are at their best. Allowing the eggplant to sweat a bit before adding it to the salad keeps it from getting too soggy later.

• 1 large green bell pepper	• 4 cloves garlic, crushed
• 1 large red bell pepper	• 2 tablespoons tomato paste
• 1 large eggplant	• ½ teaspoon kosher salt
• ½ teaspoon sea salt or kosher salt	• ½ teaspoon freshly ground black pepper
• 7 medium fresh tomatoes	• ½ teaspoon cayenne pepper
• ¼ cup coconut oil	

1. Preheat broiler to its highest setting. Place the whole peppers on a baking sheet and broil, turning often, until the skins are blackened on all sides. Place the peppers in a ziplock plastic bag, and allow them to cool.

2. Meanwhile, slice the eggplant into ½-inch strips, place in a large bowl, and sprinkle with the sea salt. Allow to sit for 20 minutes to draw out the excess water. Drain and pat dry.

3. Bring a large pot of water to a boil over high heat. Cut an X at the base of each tomato and boil for 1 minute. Immediately plunge them into an ice water bath and allow them to cool.

4. In a large skillet over medium-high heat, heat the coconut oil and then sauté the eggplant until it begins to brown, 3–4 minutes per side.

5. Rinse the peppers under cold water, and gently peel off just the ashy part of the burnt skin. Open the peppers and remove the seeds. Cut the peppers into small strips. Add peppers and garlic to the skillet with the eggplant.

6. Peel and chop the cooled tomatoes, and add to the skillet.

7. Add the tomato paste, kosher salt, black pepper, and cayenne. Bring the mixture to a boil, reduce the heat to medium, and then simmer for 30 minutes.

8. Transfer to a large bowl, cover, and chill for 2 hours before serving.

Serves 4.

Middle Eastern Bean Salad

This recipe is our version of a traditional salad from the Middle East called Balela. It's a tasty mix of garbanzo beans and black beans with tons of flavor from fresh herbs. This keeps very well, so make a large batch to eat throughout the week as a snack or a lunch.

- 2 (15-ounce) cans garbanzo beans, rinsed and drained
- 2 (15-ounce) cans black beans, rinsed and drained
- ½ cup chopped fresh mint leaves
- ½ cup chopped fresh parsley
- ½ cup chopped red onion
- 1 pint cherry tomatoes, halved
- 1 jalapeño pepper, finely chopped
- 1 clove garlic, chopped
- 5 tablespoons apple cider vinegar
- ¼ cup coconut oil
- 3 tablespoons freshly squeezed lemon juice
- ½ teaspoon salt
- ½ teaspoon freshly ground black pepper

1. In a large bowl, combine the beans, mint, parsley, onion, and tomatoes.

2. In a blender, combine the jalapeño, garlic, apple cider vinegar, coconut oil, and lemon juice, and blend on low speed until thoroughly combined.

3. Pour the dressing over the salad, and toss well to mix. Season with the salt and pepper, and then cover and chill for 2 hours before serving.

Serves 10.

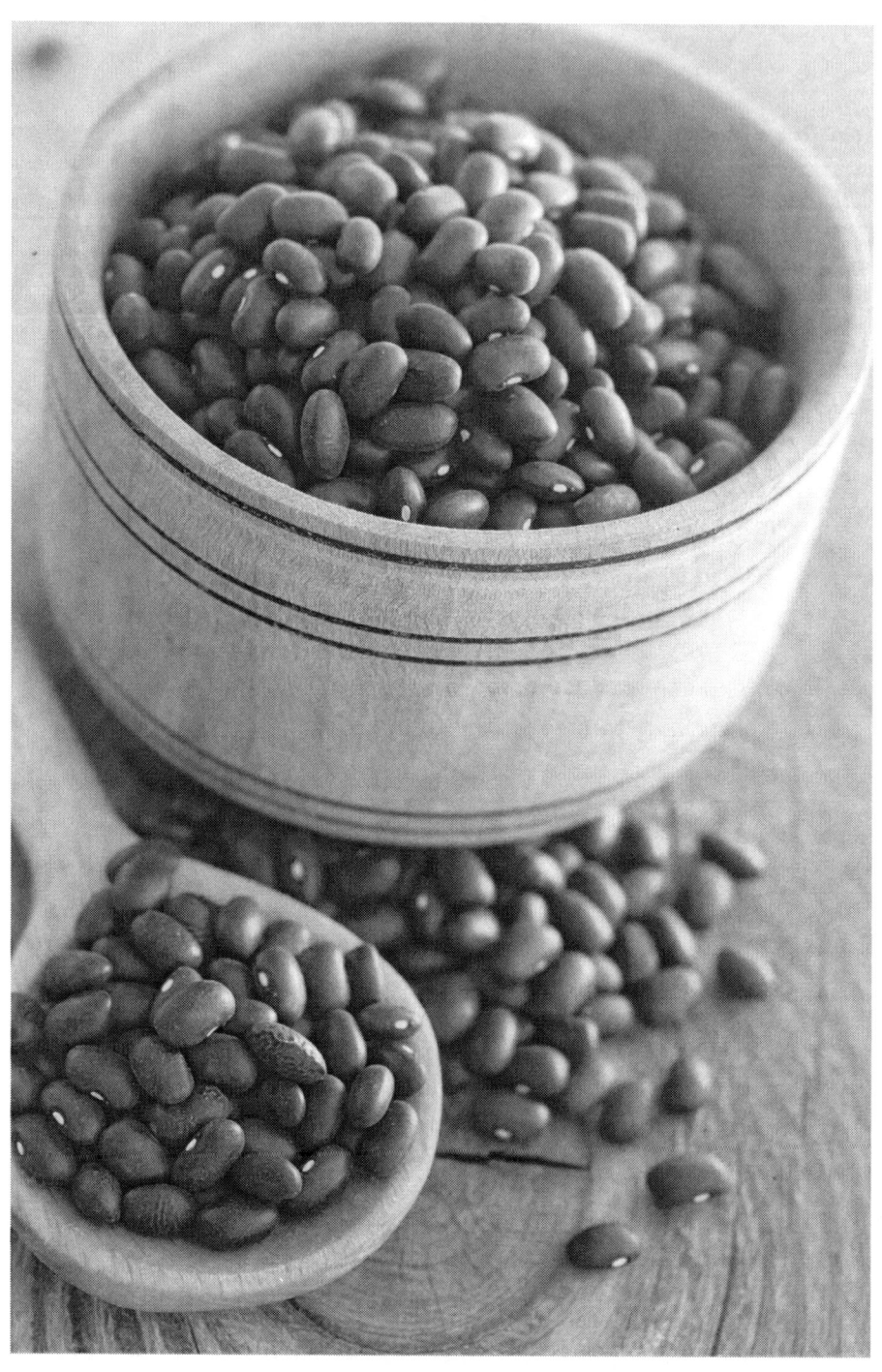

Black beans are a very rich source of several key nutrients, including iron and fiber.

8

CHINA STUDY DIET SOUPS

Spicy Black Bean Soup

Black beans are a very rich source of several key nutrients, including iron and fiber. They're also hearty and filling and make for a very inexpensive meal for those on a budget. This soup has just enough spice to make it fun, and it's great served with a green salad or some fresh fruit.

- 1 tablespoon coconut oil
- 1 large onion, chopped
- 1 stalk celery, chopped
- 2 carrots, chopped
- 4 cloves garlic, chopped
- 2 tablespoons chili powder
- 1 tablespoon ground cumin
- Pinch of freshly ground black pepper
- 4 cups vegetable broth
- 4 (15-ounce) cans black beans
- 1 (15-ounce) can whole kernel corn
- 1 (14.5-ounce) can crushed tomatoes

---

1. In a large stockpot over medium-high heat, heat the coconut oil until sizzling. Reduce the heat to medium, and add the onion, celery, carrots, garlic, chili powder, cumin, and pepper. Sauté, stirring frequently, for 3 minutes. Stir in the vegetable broth,

two cans of the beans, and the corn, and increase the heat to medium-high. Bring to a boil, and then reduce the heat again to medium.

2. In a blender, combine the tomatoes and the remaining two cans of beans, and blend until smooth. Stir the mixture into the pot and let the soup simmer for 10 minutes, stirring frequently. Ladle into bowls and serve.

Serves 10.

Curried Carrot Soup

The heady spices of curry are a beautiful accompaniment to the sweetness of carrots. This soup is rich and creamy—perfect on a cool afternoon or evening. This will keep well in the fridge for several days. Add a bit more liquid, and reheat on the stove for best results.

- 4 cups vegetable broth
- 2 teaspoons curry powder
- 1 teaspoon ground cumin
- ½ teaspoon ground cinnamon
- ½ teaspoon ground ginger
- 2 pounds carrots, peeled and chopped
- 1 (14-ounce) can coconut milk
- 1¾ cups water
- 1 teaspoon chopped fresh cilantro

1. In a large stockpot over medium-high heat, bring the vegetable broth to a boil. Stir in the curry powder, cumin, cinnamon, and ginger. Reduce the heat to medium and stir in the carrots. Simmer, stirring often, until the carrots are tender, about 15–20 minutes.

2. Remove the carrots from the pot using a slotted spoon or strainer, leaving the broth in the pot over medium heat.

3. Place enough carrots in a blender to fill it halfway, and add ¼ cup of the hot broth. Pulse a few times to break up the carrots, and then puree until smooth. Work in batches until all of the carrots have been pureed, stirring each finished batch back into the broth.

4. Add the coconut milk and water to the pot and stir. Bring the soup to a simmer and heat through. Ladle into bowls and top with cilantro before serving.

Serves 6.

Chinese Hot and Sour Soup

Hot and sour soup is a favorite dish eaten at every Chinese restaurant. This version is just as delicious as the one your favorite restaurant serves, and it's surprisingly simple to make. Most of the ingredients are pantry items, so stock up to have everything you need on hand when the craving hits.

- 1 ounce dried wood ear mushrooms
- 4 dried shiitake mushrooms
- 12 dried lily bulbs
- 2 cups hot water, divided
- ½ ounce bamboo fungus
- Salt to taste
- 3 tablespoons soy sauce
- 5 tablespoons rice vinegar
- 4 tablespoons cornstarch, divided
- 1 (8-ounce) container firm tofu, thinly sliced
- 1 quart vegetable broth
- ¾ teaspoon ground white pepper
- ½ teaspoon ground black pepper
- ¼ teaspoon crushed red pepper flakes
- ½ tablespoon chili oil
- ½ tablespoon sesame oil
- 1 green onion, sliced

1. Place the wood ear mushrooms, shiitake mushrooms, and lily bulbs in a small bowl, and cover with 1½ cups of the hot water. Allow them to soak for 20 minutes, or until the mushrooms are plump and rehydrated. Drain, reserving the liquid. Trim the stems from the mushrooms, and cut them into thin strips. Cut each lily bulb in half.

2. In another small bowl, soak the bamboo fungus in ¼ cup of the hot water with a sprinkling of salt. Soak for about 20 minutes, or until rehydrated. Drain and chop the fungus, and set aside.

3. In a medium bowl, whisk together the soy sauce, rice vinegar, and 1 tablespoon of the cornstarch. Place half of the tofu into this mixture and toss to coat.

4. In a medium saucepan, combine the reserved mushroom broth with the vegetable broth. Bring to a boil over medium-high heat; then add the mushrooms and lily bulbs. Reduce the heat to low and simmer for 5 minutes. Season with the white and black pepper and red pepper flakes.

5. In a small bowl, whisk together the remaining 3 tablespoons cornstarch and the remaining ¼ cup hot water. Whisk into the broth mixture until slightly thickened.

6. Stir both the tofu with soy sauce and plain tofu into the saucepan. Increase the heat to medium-high, and return the soup to a boil. Stir in the bamboo fungus, chili oil, and sesame oil. Garnish with the green onion and serve.

Serves 6.

Creamy Corn Chowder

Corn chowder is one of those classic dishes that everyone is happy to find waiting at the table. This version is creamy, rich, and delicious, and very simple to make. By all means, use fresh corn when in season, but frozen kernels work very well and make this soup available in the cooler months.

- 2 teaspoons coconut oil
- 1 medium onion, finely chopped
- 3 stalks celery, finely chopped
- 3 carrots, finely chopped
- 4 pounds red potatoes, scrubbed and finely chopped
- 1 medium head cauliflower, cut into bite-sized pieces
- 2 bay leaves
- ½ teaspoon dried thyme
- ½ teaspoon dried tarragon
- 2 quarts vegetable broth
- 8 cups fresh corn, divided
- 1 cup cashews
- ½ cup nutritional yeast
- 1 teaspoon salt
- ½ teaspoon freshly ground black pepper

1. Heat the coconut oil in a large soup pot over medium heat. Add the onion, celery, and carrots and sauté, stirring frequently, for 5–7 minutes, or until slightly tender.

2. Add the potatoes, cauliflower, bay leaves, thyme, and tarragon, and cook for 5 more minutes.

3. Add the vegetable broth and 6 cups of the corn to the pot, increase the heat to medium-high, and bring to a boil. Reduce the heat to low and simmer for 35–40 minutes, or until the vegetables are tender. Remove the bay leaves.

4. Combine the remaining 2 cups of corn, the cashews, and the nutritional yeast in a blender, and add several large spoonfuls of the hot broth. Working in two batches as needed (fill the blender no more than halfway), blend until smooth.

5. Stir the corn-cashew puree into the soup and heat through. Season with the salt and pepper, and then ladle into bowls to serve.

Serves 8.

Hearty Split Pea Soup

This soup is wonderfully rich and satisfying. This is a great dish to let simmer on the stove all day. Just keep adding more water occasionally if it begins to get too dry. This soup tastes better the second day, so make it ahead or just be sure to hide a secret container of leftovers for later.

- 1 tablespoon coconut oil
- 1 large onion, chopped
- 1 bay leaf
- 3 cloves garlic, chopped
- 2 cups dried split peas
- ½ cup barley
- 1½ teaspoons salt
- 7½ cups water
- 3 carrots, chopped
- 3 stalks celery, chopped
- 3 medium russet potatoes, diced
- ½ cup chopped fresh parsley
- ½ teaspoon dried basil
- ½ teaspoon dried thyme
- ½ teaspoon freshly ground black pepper

1. In a large stockpot, heat the coconut oil over medium-high heat. Add the onion, bay leaf, and garlic and sauté for 5 minutes, or just until the onions are translucent.

2. Add the split peas, barley, salt, and water. Bring the mixture to a boil, and then reduce the heat to low. Cover and simmer for 2 hours, stirring occasionally and adding more water if needed.

3. Add the carrots, celery, potatoes, parsley, basil, thyme, and pepper. Simmer for about 1 more hour, or until the peas and vegetables are tender. Ladle into bowls and serve.

Serves 10.

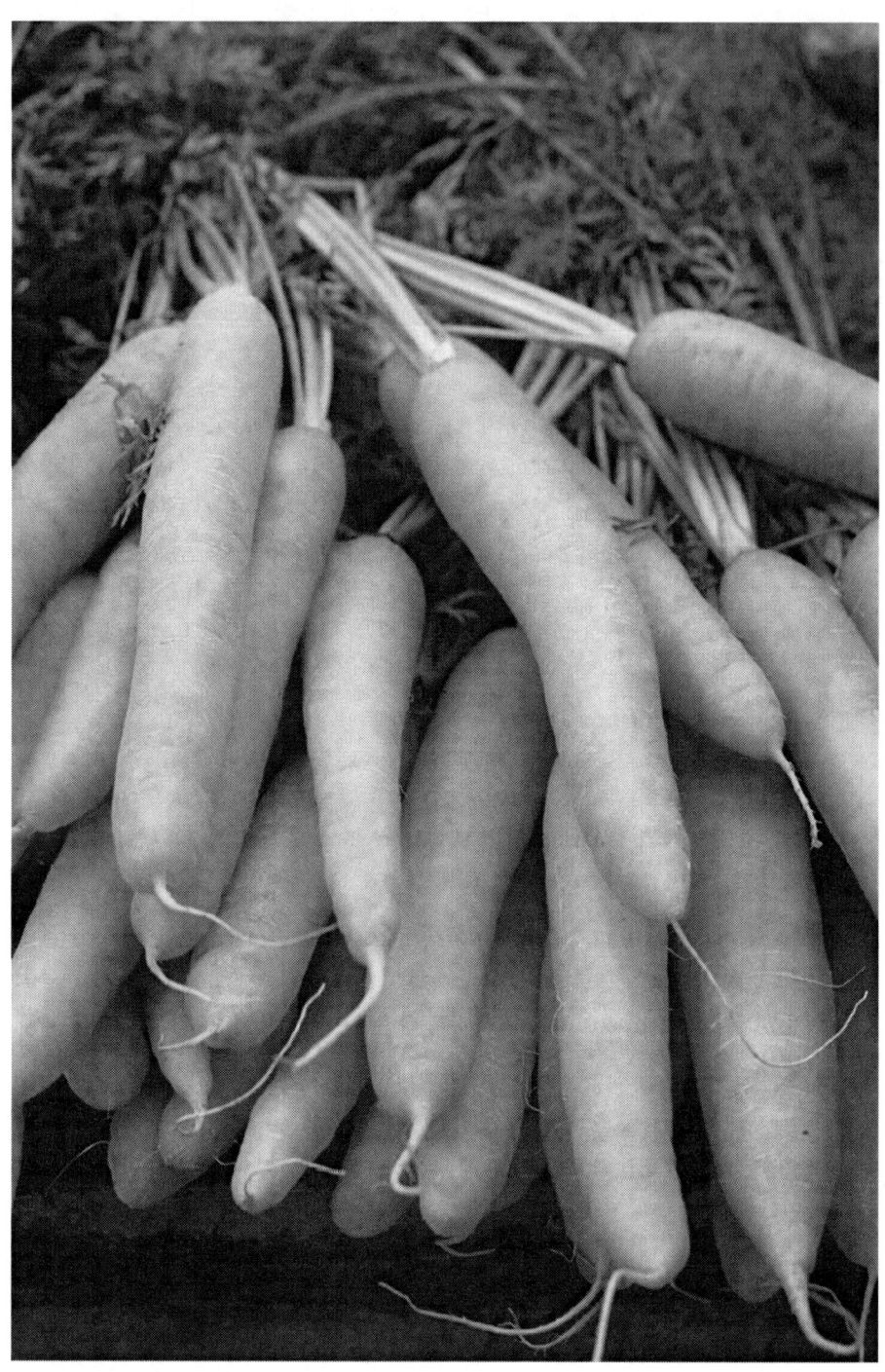

Carrots are beautifully sweet on their own.

Chunky Vegetable Soup

This is no thin, unsatisfying vegetable soup. It's chock-full of lots of chunky vegetables and is loaded with flavor. Served with a good bread and fresh fruit for dessert, this is a complete and nutritious meal that will satisfy you throughout the day.

- 2 tablespoons coconut oil
- ½ medium onion, chopped
- 3 stalks celery, chopped
- 2 cloves garlic, minced
- 4 cups vegetable broth
- 1 (15-ounce) can tomato sauce
- 4 carrots, peeled and cut into ¼-inch-thick coins
- 2 baking potatoes, cut into bite-sized pieces
- 1 cup fresh or frozen corn kernels
- 1 cup frozen shelled edamame
- 1 cup sliced okra
- 1 cup roughly chopped kale
- 1 teaspoon salt
- 1 teaspoon freshly ground black pepper

1. In a large stockpot over medium heat, heat the coconut oil until melted.

2. Stir in the onion and celery and sauté for about 5 minutes, or just until softened. Stir in the garlic and cook, stirring frequently, until very fragrant, about 2–3 minutes.

3. Add the vegetable broth and tomato sauce to the pot, and simmer for about 10 minutes.

4. Stir in the carrots and potatoes and simmer until the carrots are tender, about 10 more minutes. Stir in the corn, edamame, okra, and kale, and continue to simmer until the okra is tender, about 5 minutes.

5. Season with the salt and pepper, ladle into bowls, and serve.

Serves 10.

Garlicky Asparagus Soup

This soup is easy to make, beautiful to look at, and deliciously different to eat. The sweet, nutty flavor of the asparagus is balanced by the tang of a healthy dose of fresh garlic. This will make four light first-course portions or serve two as a main-course soup.

- 1 tablespoon coconut oil
- 5 cloves fresh garlic, thinly sliced
- 4 scallions, coarsely chopped
- 1½ pounds asparagus, trimmed and coarsely chopped
- 3½ cups vegetable broth
- ½ teaspoon salt
- ¼ teaspoon ground white pepper

1. Heat the coconut oil in a saucepan over medium heat. Add the garlic and scallions, and cook just until the garlic is golden, about 3 minutes.

2. Stir in the asparagus and sauté until just slightly tender, about 3 more minutes.

3. Pour in the vegetable broth, increase the heat to medium-high, and bring to a boil. Reduce the heat to medium-low and simmer until the asparagus is tender, about 10 minutes. Remove the pan from the heat and allow the soup to cool for about 15 minutes.

4. Pour the soup into a blender, filling it no more than halfway. Work in batches as needed. Puree the soup until smooth.

5. Transfer the soup back to the saucepan over medium heat to warm it through. Season with the salt and white pepper, ladle into bowls, and serve.

Serves 2–4.

Chunky Vegetarian Chili

Even the most diehard carnivore will love this spicy, hearty chili. It's loaded with flavor, packed with vegetables, and has enough kick to please any true chili lover. This is especially good reheated over a couple of days, so make a big batch and take the leftovers to work.

- 1 tablespoon coconut oil
- ½ medium red onion, chopped
- 2 bay leaves
- 2 tablespoons dried oregano
- 1 tablespoon salt
- 1 teaspoon ground cumin
- 2 stalks celery, chopped
- 2 green bell peppers, chopped
- 2 jalapeño peppers, chopped
- 3 cloves garlic, chopped
- 2 (4-ounce) cans chopped green chili peppers, drained
- 2 (12-ounce) packages crumbled tofu
- 3 (28-ounce) cans whole peeled tomatoes, crushed
- ¼ cup chili powder
- 1 tablespoon freshly ground black pepper
- 1 (15-ounce) can kidney beans, drained
- 1 (15-ounce) can garbanzo beans, drained
- 1 (15-ounce) can black beans, with liquid
- 1 (12-ounce) package frozen corn

1. Heat the coconut oil in a large stockpot over medium heat. Add the onion, bay leaves, oregano, salt, and cumin. Sauté until the onions are tender, and then stir in the celery, bell peppers, jalapeños, garlic, and chili peppers. Sauté for 2 minutes, stirring frequently.

2. Stir in the tofu crumbles. Reduce the heat to low, cover, and simmer for 5 minutes.

3. Add the tomatoes to the pot and season with the chili powder and black pepper. Stir in all of the beans. Increase the heat to medium-high and bring to a boil, reduce the heat to low, and simmer for 45 minutes.

4. Stir in the corn and cook until heated through. Ladle into bowls and serve.

Serves 8.

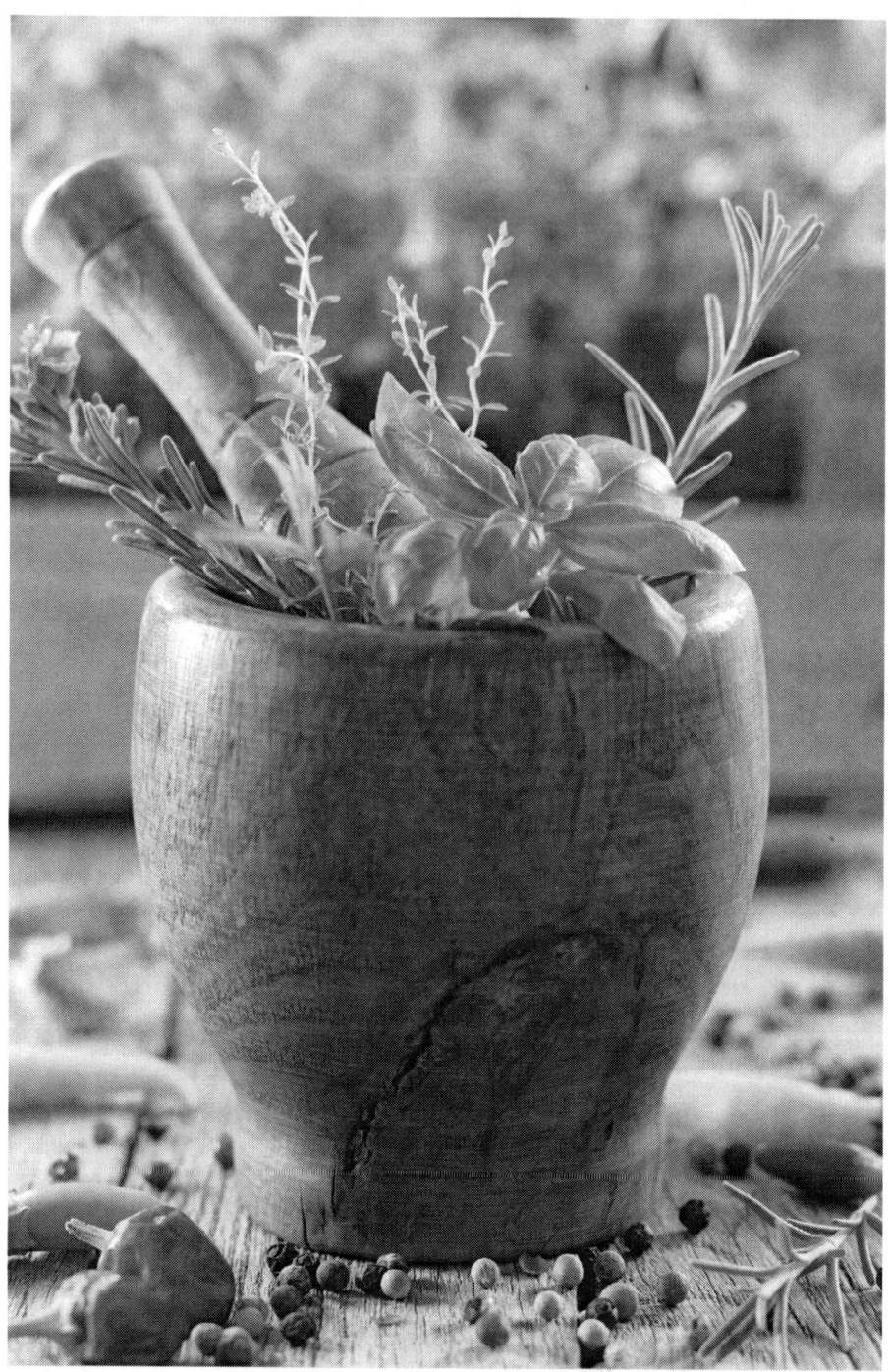

Herbs contain a wide array of essential minerals and vitamins. Remember that fresh herbs pack the most nutritional value.

Rich Homemade Vegetable Stock

A good vegetable stock is invaluable as a base for soups, stews, and sauces. The canned variety available in stores pales in comparison to the depth of flavor in this easy-to-make stock. The nuanced layers come from roasting the vegetables, which brings out all of their natural goodness.

- 1 whole head of garlic
- 4 carrots, cut into chunks
- 4 stalks celery, cut into chunks
- 3 medium onions, cut into chunks
- 1 green bell pepper, quartered
- 1 large tomato, quartered
- ¼ cup coconut oil
- ½ teaspoon salt
- ½ teaspoon freshly ground black pepper
- 2 quarts water
- 1½ teaspoons dried thyme
- 1½ teaspoons dried parsley
- 2 bay leaves

1. Preheat oven to 400 degrees F, and line a baking sheet with aluminum foil.

2. Slice the top from the entire head of garlic. Arrange the garlic, carrots, celery, onions, bell pepper, and tomato in a single layer on the baking sheet. Drizzle the coconut oil over the vegetables, and toss with your hands to coat. Season with the salt and pepper.

3. Roast the vegetables, stirring every 15 minutes or so, until they're tender and browned, about 1 hour.

4. In a large stockpot over medium-high heat, combine the water, thyme, parsley, and bay leaves. Squeeze the roasted garlic into the pot and throw away the papery husk. Add the rest of the roasted vegetables to the pot and bring to a boil. Reduce the heat to low and simmer for 1½ hours.

5. Strain and discard the solids, and allow the stock to cool to room temperature before storing in the refrigerator in an airtight container for up to 2 weeks.

Makes about 2 quarts.

Simple Minestrone

Minestrone is a wonderful soup. It is filled with the flavors of summer and garden-fresh vegetables. The herbs and seasonings are classic Italian, and this version of the recipe is completely compatible with the China Study, without sacrificing any of the dish's delicious essence.

- 3 tablespoons coconut oil
- 1 leek, thinly sliced
- 2 carrots, chopped
- 1 medium zucchini, thinly sliced
- 4 ounces green beans, cut into 1-inch pieces
- 2 stalks celery, thinly sliced
- 6 cups vegetable stock
- 1 pound fresh tomatoes, chopped
- 1 tablespoon chopped fresh thyme
- 1 (15-ounce) can cannellini beans, with liquid
- ½ teaspoon salt
- ¼ teaspoon freshly ground black pepper

1. Melt the coconut oil in a large saucepan over medium-high heat. Add the leek, carrots, zucchini, green beans, and celery. Reduce the heat to low, cover the pot, and simmer for 15 minutes, stirring occasionally.

2. Add the vegetable stock, tomatoes, and thyme to the pot. Increase the heat to medium-high, and bring the soup to a boil. Reduce the heat to low, cover, and simmer for 30 more minutes.

3. Stir in the beans and continue cooking for 10 more minutes. Season with the salt and pepper, ladle into bowls, and serve.

Serves 4.

Super Green Gazpacho

Green plants are filled with many of the most healthful and essential antioxidants. This has led to the popularity of "green" drinks. This no-cook recipe delivers the same level of nutrition in a flavorful and elegant soup that's perfect for hot weather.

- 2 cups diced honeydew melon
- 1 seedless English cucumber, peeled and chopped
- 1 small red onion, finely diced
- 1 avocado, diced
- 1 jalapeño pepper, seeded and finely chopped
- 1 clove garlic, chopped
- ¼ cup white balsamic vinegar
- 1 tablespoon freshly squeezed lime juice
- ¼ teaspoon salt
- ¼ teaspoon freshly ground black pepper

1. In a food processor or blender, combine all of the ingredients. Work in two batches as needed. Blend until the gazpacho is very smooth and a uniform pale green color.

2. Chill for at least 2 hours in a covered container before serving.

Serves 2.

Creamy Tomato Soup

The canned tomato soup from the store is thickened with cornstarch and milk. It's also loaded with sodium and sugar. This version uses soft tofu in place of the milk, lending it a wonderful silkiness and also giving this soup a healthy portion of protein.

- 1 tablespoon coconut oil
- 4 cups diced tomatoes
- ¼ cup chopped onion
- 1 clove garlic, chopped
- 1 (14-ounce) package soft tofu
- 1 (6-ounce) can tomato paste
- 1 teaspoon honey
- ½ teaspoon salt
- ¼ teaspoon freshly ground black pepper

1. In a medium saucepan, melt the coconut oil over medium heat. Add the tomatoes, onion, and garlic, and sauté for about 5 minutes, or until the onions are translucent.

2. In a blender, puree the tofu, tomato paste, and honey until very smooth.

3. Add the tofu mixture to the pan and heat until warmed through.

4. Season the soup with the salt and pepper, and add water as needed to achieve the desired consistency. Ladle into bowls and serve.

Serves 6.

Orchard Peach Soup

If at all possible, buy locally grown, tree-ripened peaches for this recipe. These will be at their absolute peak of flavor, rather than picked long before they're ripe. In a pinch, you can buy frozen peaches to make this soup, or better yet, buy fresh peaches in season and then can or freeze them yourself to use later.

- 4 cloves garlic
- 1 tablespoon coconut oil
- 2¼ cups peeled and chopped fresh peaches
- ½ cup diced yellow onion
- ¼ cup honey
- 1 tablespoon mild curry powder
- ⅛ teaspoon ground turmeric
- ¼ cup apple cider
- 1 cup vegetable stock or broth
- ½ cup coconut milk
- ¼ teaspoon salt
- ¼ teaspoon freshly ground black pepper

1. Preheat oven to 275 degrees F. Line a baking sheet with aluminum foil, and roast the garlic for about 30 minutes, or until golden but not brown.

2. Heat the coconut oil in a medium saucepan over medium heat. Gently sauté the peaches and onion until softened, about 10 minutes. Season with honey, curry powder, turmeric, and roasted garlic. Reduce the heat to medium-low and cook until caramelized, about 30 minutes.

3. Deglaze the pan with the apple cider, scraping up any browned bits on the bottom of the pan. Stir in the vegetable stock.

4. Transfer the soup to a blender or food processor and puree. Work in two batches as needed. Strain the soup through a fine sieve.

5. Stir in the coconut milk and season with the salt and pepper. This soup can be served at room temperature or reheated to serve warm.

Serves 4.

Amazing Autumn Kale Stew

This hearty stew is perfect for cool fall evenings or lunch on a winter day. Kale is one of the dark leafy greens that is at its best when hit with a touch of frost. This makes it an excellent choice in winter when other greens are imported or unavailable.

- 2 tablespoons coconut oil
- 1 medium yellow onion, chopped
- 2 tablespoons chopped garlic
- 1 bunch kale, stems removed, chopped
- 2 quarts water
- 6 cubes vegetable bouillon
- 1 (15-ounce) can diced tomatoes
- 6 small white potatoes, peeled and diced
- 2 (15-ounce) cans cannellini beans, with liquid
- 1 tablespoon Italian seasoning
- 2 tablespoons dried parsley
- ½ teaspoon salt
- ¼ teaspoon freshly ground black pepper

1. In a large stockpot, melt the coconut oil over medium heat. Add the onion and garlic, and cook just until soft, about 3 minutes. Stir in the kale and cook until just wilted, about 2 minutes.

2. Add the water, vegetable bouillon, tomatoes, potatoes, beans, Italian seasoning, and parsley. Simmer for 25 minutes, or until the potatoes are tender.

3. Season with the salt and pepper, ladle into bowls, and serve.

Serves 8.

Savory Lima Bean Soup

This soup is surprisingly satisfying. The flavor will intensify if left overnight, so make it a day ahead to enjoy it at its best. Experiment with whatever other vegetables are in season, and add them to the soup to vary the flavor, as lima beans are mild enough to work with any of them.

- 1 gallon water, divided
- 1 pound dry lima beans
- 2 tablespoons coconut oil
- 5 carrots, peeled and chopped
- 2 stalks celery, chopped
- 1 leek, white only, chopped
- 2 tablespoons chopped shallots
- 4 cubes vegetable bouillon

1. In a large saucepan, bring 1 quart water to a boil over high heat. Add the lima beans and boil for about 3 minutes. Remove from the heat, cover, and allow the beans to sit for 1–2 hours, or until softened. Drain and rinse until the water runs clear. Drain well.

2. In a large pot, melt the coconut oil over medium-high heat and sauté the carrots, celery, leeks, and shallots until tender, about 5 minutes. Add the lima beans, and sauté for 3 more minutes.

3. Meanwhile, in a small saucepan, bring 1 quart water to a boil. Add the vegetable bouillon and stir until dissolved. Add this broth to the soup pot.

4. Add another 8 cups water to the pot, and allow the soup to simmer over low heat for 10 minutes. Ladle into bowls and serve.

Serves 8.

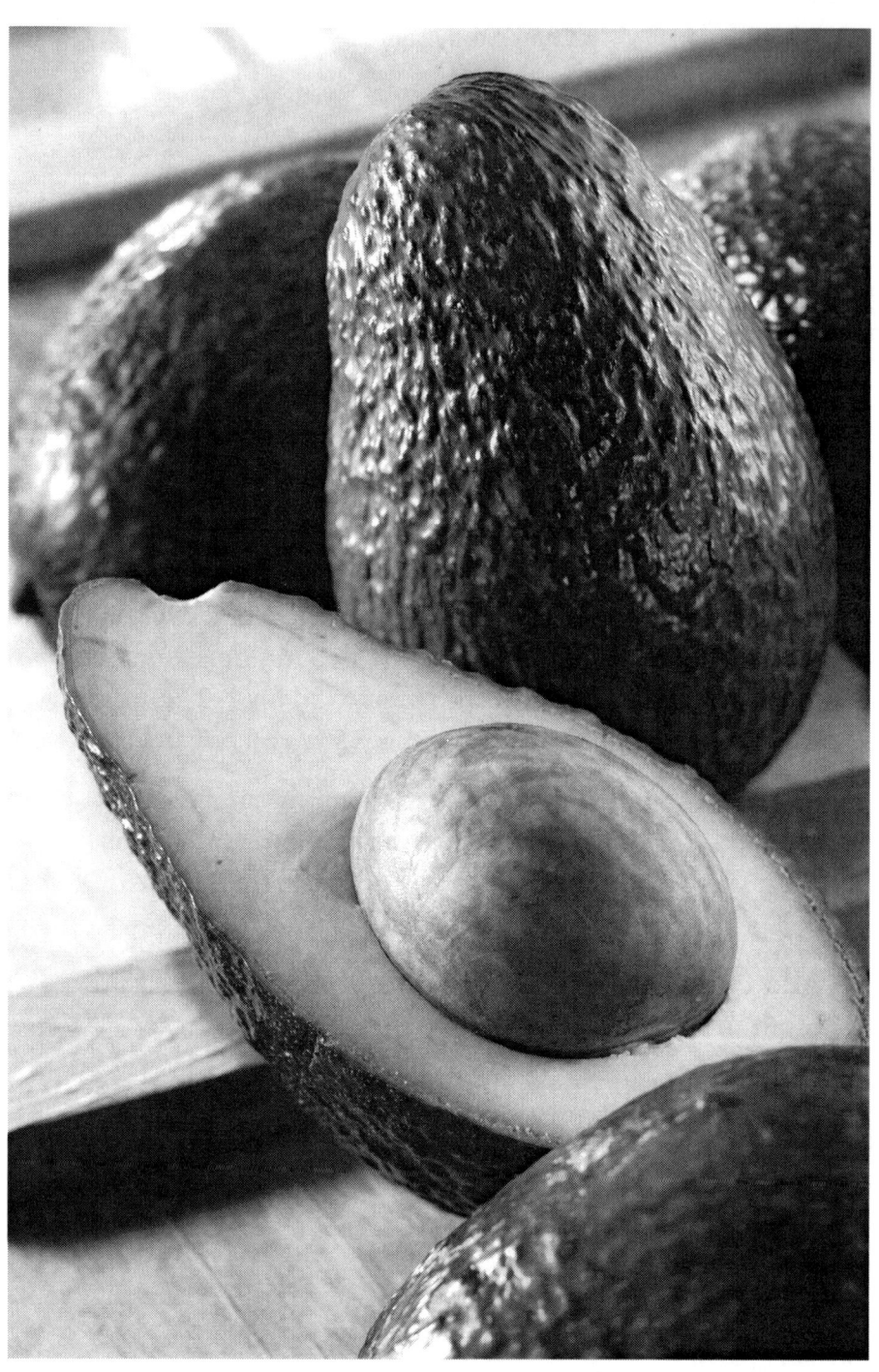

Plant-based fats such as avocado oil are rich in antioxidants.

9

CHINA STUDY DIET DINNERS

Spicy Potato Curry

The spice of a good curry dish is warming, satisfying, and layered with nuances that have a lot more to offer than just heat. This recipe is loaded with potatoes, vegetables, and other goodies in a creamy, spicy sauce that begs to be savored to the last drop.

- 4 medium potatoes, peeled and cubed
- 2 tablespoons coconut oil
- 1 yellow onion, diced
- 3 cloves garlic, minced
- 4 teaspoons curry powder
- 4 teaspoons garam masala
- 2 teaspoons salt, divided
- 2 teaspoons ground cumin
- 1½ teaspoons cayenne pepper
- ½ teaspoon minced fresh ginger
- 1½ cups diced fresh tomatoes
- 1 (15-ounce) can garbanzo beans, rinsed and drained
- 1 (12-ounce) package frozen peas, thawed and drained
- 1 (14-ounce) can coconut milk

1. Place the potatoes in a large stockpot and cover with water. Add 1 teaspoon salt and bring to a boil over high heat. Reduce the

heat to medium-low, cover, and simmer for about 15 minutes, or just until tender. Drain the potatoes and allow them to dry for about 5 minutes.

2. Meanwhile, heat the coconut oil in a large skillet over medium heat. Stir in the onion and garlic and sauté just until the onion is translucent, about 5 minutes. Add the curry powder, garam masala, remaining 1 teaspoon of salt, cumin, cayenne, and ginger. Cook for 2 more minutes.

3. Add the potatoes, tomatoes, beans, peas, and coconut milk. Increase the heat to medium-high and simmer for 5–10 minutes. Ladle into bowls and serve.

Serves 6.

Black Beans and Quinoa

This dish is a riff on the more traditional South and Central American classic dish of black beans and rice. Quinoa is a great source of both protein and healthy fats, two nutrients that can be hard to get enough of on a strictly plant-based diet.

- 1 teaspoon coconut oil
- 1 medium onion, chopped
- 3 cloves garlic, chopped
- ¾ cup uncooked quinoa
- 1½ cups vegetable broth
- 1 teaspoon ground cumin
- ¼ teaspoon cayenne pepper
- ¼ teaspoon salt
- ¼ teaspoon freshly ground black pepper
- 1 cup fresh or frozen corn kernels
- 2 (15-ounce) cans black beans, rinsed and drained
- ½ cup chopped fresh cilantro

1. In a saucepan over medium-high heat, heat the coconut oil. Add the onion and garlic, and sauté for about 5 minutes, or until lightly browned.

2. Stir the quinoa into the pan and add the vegetable broth. Season with the cumin, cayenne, salt, and pepper. Bring the mixture to a boil, cover, reduce the heat to low, and simmer for 20 minutes.

3. Stir in the corn and simmer for 5 more minutes. Stir in the black beans and half of the cilantro, reserving some for garnish. Heat thoroughly.

4. Ladle the soup into bowls, garnish with cilantro, and serve.

Serves 8.

Grilled Tofu Kabobs with Red Pepper Sauce

Tofu is such a versatile ingredient; firm tofu easily stands in for many meats and is a great boon to a plant-based diet. In this recipe, the tofu acts much like chicken breast and absorbs the flavors of the sauce and vegetables beautifully.

- 1 (8-ounce) container extra-firm tofu
- 1 medium zucchini, cut into large chunks
- 1 red bell pepper, cut into large chunks
- 10 large mushrooms
- ¼ cup soy sauce
- 2 tablespoons red chili garlic sauce
- 2 tablespoons coconut oil, melted
- ¼ cup diced onion
- 1 jalapeño pepper, diced
- ½ teaspoon freshly ground black pepper
- Metal or bamboo skewers

1. Drain the tofu very well and pat dry with paper towels. Cut it into ½-inch chunks.

2. Place the tofu, zucchini, bell pepper, and mushrooms in a large bowl.

3. In a small bowl, combine the soy sauce, red chili sauce, melted coconut oil, onion, jalapeño, and black pepper, and whisk until well blended.

4. Pour the marinade over the tofu and vegetables. Toss lightly to coat. Cover and allow the vegetables and tofu to marinate for at least 1 hour in the refrigerator.

5. Preheat the grill to medium-high heat, and lightly oil the rack.

6. Alternate the tofu and vegetables on the skewers. Grill each skewer for 10 minutes, turning several times. Reserve any remaining marinade to use as a dipping sauce.

Serves 8.

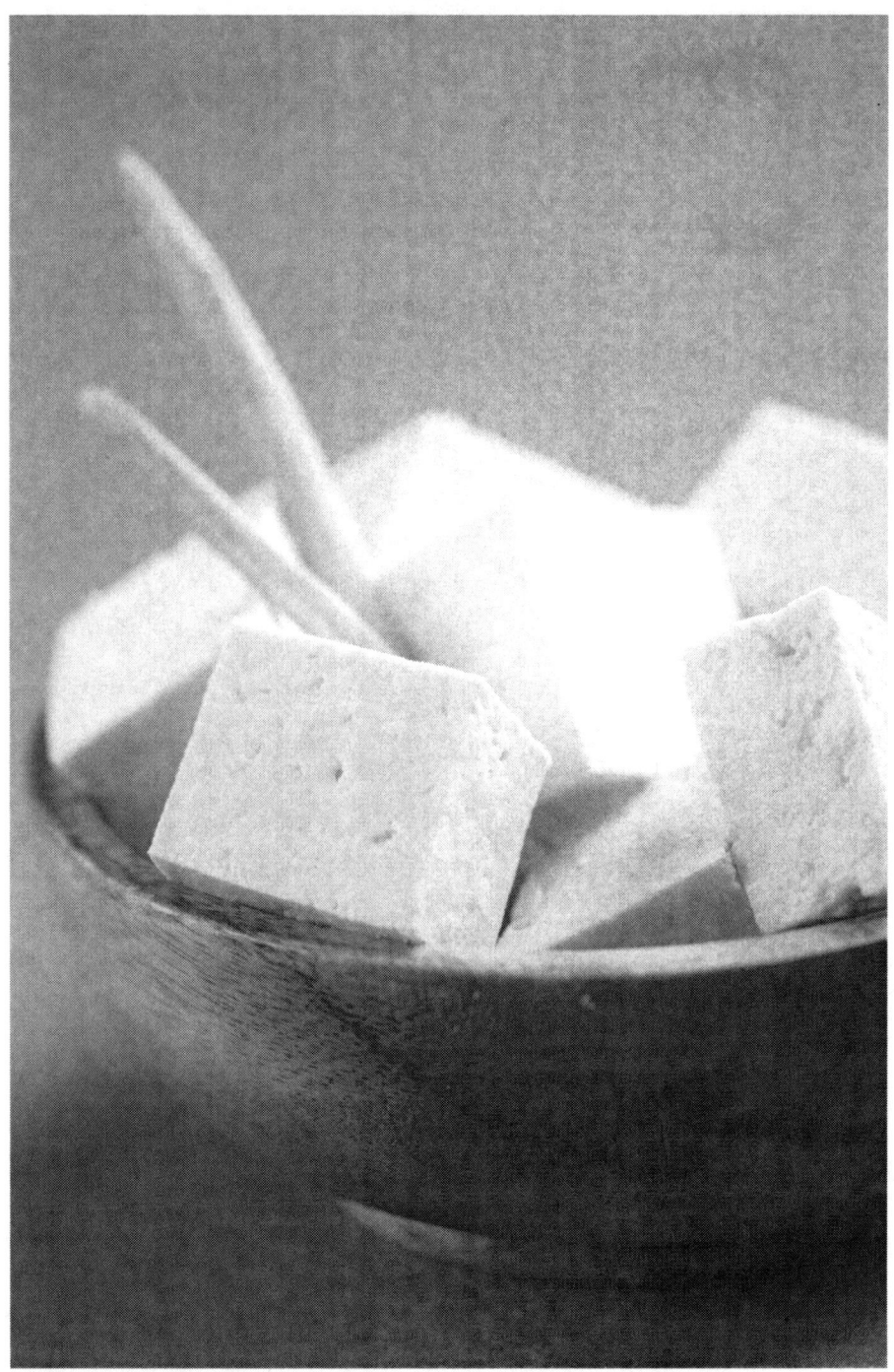

Tofu is a versatile ingredient. Firm tofu easily stands in for many meats and is a great boon to a plant-based diet.

Thai-Style Grilled Tofu Steaks

The classic Thai flavors of cilantro and lime marry beautifully in this dish. Don't skip the steps of weighting and pressing the tofu to remove the excess water; the tofu needs to be very dry to get a good sear and a nicely grilled color. Note that the tofu needs to marinate for at least 3 hours or ideally overnight for best results.

- 1 (14-ounce) package firm tofu
- ¼ cup freshly squeezed lime juice
- 1 tablespoon coconut oil
- 5 tablespoons chopped fresh cilantro
- 2 cloves garlic, chopped
- 2 teaspoons chili powder
- ½ teaspoon cayenne pepper
- ½ teaspoon salt
- ¼ teaspoon freshly ground black pepper

1. Place the tofu on a plate and cover with a small cutting board or baking pan. Set a 2- to 3-pound hand weight or a few canned goods on top to weigh down the tofu. Let the tofu sit for 20 minutes, draining off any accumulated liquid as needed. Drain the tofu well, pat dry with paper towels, and slice into 4 "steaks."

2. In a small bowl, whisk together the lime juice, coconut oil, cilantro, garlic, chili powder, cayenne, salt, and pepper.

3. Brush the marinade onto the tofu, cover with plastic wrap, and marinate in the refrigerator overnight or for at least 3 hours.

4. Preheat the grill to medium heat, and lightly oil the rack.

5. Grill the tofu for 10–15 minutes, turning frequently, until nicely colored and heated through.

Serves 4.

Moroccan Vegetable Curry

This curry is loaded with fresh vegetables, garbanzo beans, and cashews. It has lots of texture, has even more flavor, and makes a great dish for a buffet or potluck. Feel free to substitute different vegetables depending on what's in season or on hand.

- 6 tablespoons coconut oil, divided
- 1 sweet potato, peeled and diced
- 1 medium eggplant, diced
- 1 cup cauliflower florets, broken into small pieces
- 1 red bell pepper, chopped
- 2 carrots, thinly sliced
- 1 large onion, chopped
- 3 cloves garlic, minced
- 1 tablespoon curry powder
- ¾ tablespoon sea salt
- 1 teaspoon ground turmeric
- 1 teaspoon ground cinnamon
- ¾ teaspoon cayenne pepper
- 1 (15-ounce) can garbanzo beans, drained
- 1 medium zucchini, sliced
- ¼ cup raw cashew halves
- 2 tablespoons raisins
- 1 cup orange juice
- 10 ounces fresh spinach leaves or frozen spinach, thawed

1. In a large stockpot, heat 3 tablespoons of the coconut oil over medium-high heat. Add the sweet potato, eggplant, cauliflower, bell pepper, carrots, and onion, and sauté for 5 minutes, stirring frequently.

2. Meanwhile, in a medium saucepan add the remaining 3 tablespoons of coconut oil, garlic, curry powder, salt, turmeric, cinnamon, and cayenne, and sauté over medium-low heat for 3 minutes.

3. Add the garlic mixture to the vegetables. Stir in the beans, zucchini, cashews, raisins, and orange juice. Cover and simmer for 20 minutes.

4. Stir in the spinach and cook until heated through.

Serves 6.

Summertime Stove-Top Ratatouille

Ratatouille is a classic dish from southern France that makes the most of summer vegetables, allowing them to shine on their own without a lot of interference. It's wonderful by itself or served over quinoa, brown rice, or another grain.

- ½ cup coconut oil, divided
- 2 medium onions, sliced into thin rings
- 3 cloves garlic, minced
- 2 medium zucchini, cubed
- 2 medium yellow squash, cubed
- 2 green bell peppers, seeded and cubed
- 1 yellow bell pepper, diced
- 1 red bell pepper, chopped
- 1 medium eggplant, cubed
- ½ teaspoon salt
- ¼ teaspoon freshly ground black pepper
- 1 bay leaf
- 4 sprigs fresh thyme
- 4 plum tomatoes, chopped
- 2 tablespoons chopped fresh parsley

1. In a large stockpot over medium-high heat, heat 1½ tablespoons of the coconut oil. Add the onions and garlic, and sauté until soft, about 5 minutes. Remove from the heat.

2. In a large skillet, heat another 1½ tablespoons of the coconut oil, and sauté the zucchini in batches until lightly golden on both sides. Add the zucchini to the pot with the onions.

3. Sauté all the remaining vegetables (through the eggplant) in this manner, one kind at a time, adding 1½ tablespoons coconut oil to the skillet with each batch. Add each sautéed vegetable, one kind at a time, to the stockpot.

4. Season the vegetable mixture with the salt and pepper. Add the bay leaf and thyme, and cover. Bring to a simmer over medium heat and cook for 15–20 minutes.

5. Add the tomatoes and parsley to the pot, and simmer for 10–15 more minutes, stirring occasionally. Remove the bay leaf and serve.

Serves 4.

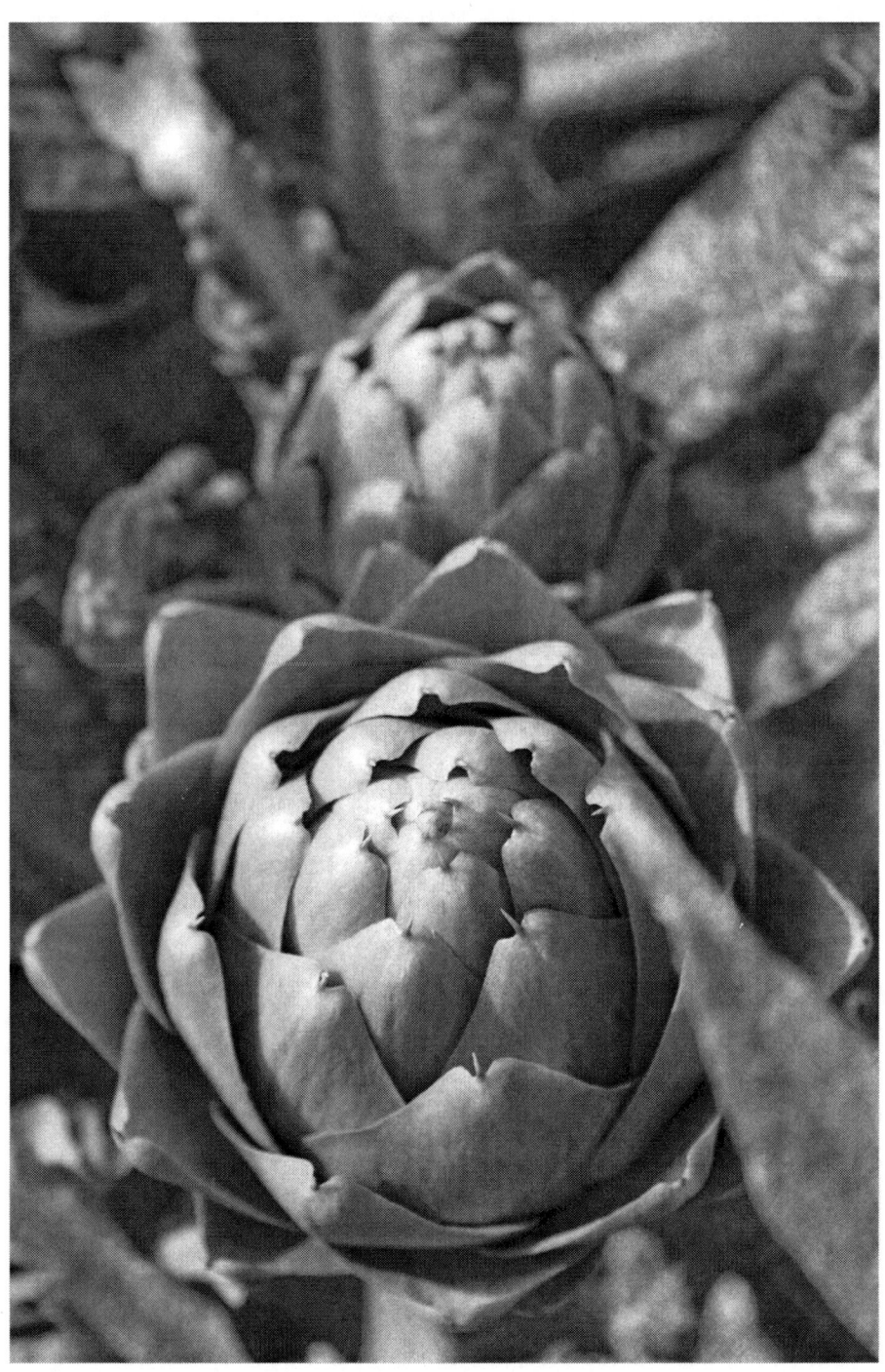

Artichokes are higher in antioxidants than any other vegetable.

Flavorful Black Bean Burgers

Black beans are a great stand-in for ground meat in vegetarian burgers. They tend to hang onto their moisture better than many other substitutes, and the appearance is closer to that of beef than with other beans.

- 1 tablespoon ground flaxseed
- 3 tablespoons water
- 1 (15-ounce) can black beans, drained and mashed
- ¼ cup panko bread crumbs
- 1 clove garlic, minced
- ½ teaspoon salt
- ½ tablespoon Worcestershire sauce
- ¼ teaspoon liquid smoke flavoring
- Coconut oil

1. Whisk the flaxseed and water together in a small bowl. Let stand for about 5 minutes, or until thickened.

2. In a medium bowl, stir together the flaxseed mixture, black beans, panko, garlic, salt, Worcestershire, and liquid smoke until well blended.

3. Form the mixture into four patties and chill until set, about 30 minutes.

4. Melt 1 or 2 tablespoons of coconut oil (or more) in a skillet over medium-high heat. Sauté the bean patties for 5 minutes on each side.

5. Serve on whole grain rolls or in a lettuce wrap.

Serves 4.

Quinoa-Stuffed Butternut Squash

Butternut squash is a delicious and filling main dish when stuffed with a fragrant mix of quinoa and seasonings. You can also make this dish with acorn squash or other varieties of winter squash. Follow the package directions for preparing the quinoa.

- 1 butternut squash, halved and seeded
- ½ cup cooked quinoa
- 6 brussels sprouts, trimmed and quartered
- 1 medium carrot, julienned
- ½ (15.5-ounce) can garbanzo beans, rinsed and drained
- ¼ cup coconut milk
- 3 tablespoons tamari, plus additional for serving
- ½ teaspoon ground turmeric
- 2 cloves garlic, minced

1. Preheat oven to 400 degrees F.

2. Place the butternut squash cut sides down in a baking dish, and add water to fill the dish 1 inch deep. Cover tightly with foil and bake for 1 hour, or until the flesh is fork tender. Keep warm.

3. Meanwhile, in a large skillet over medium-high heat, sauté the quinoa, brussels sprouts, carrots, and garbanzo beans.

4. In a small bowl, stir together the coconut milk, tamari, turmeric, and garlic, and add to the skillet, tossing to coat.

5. Cover the skillet and simmer for 20 minutes, or until the vegetables are tender.

6. Spoon the mixture into the squash. Serve with additional tamari if desired.

Serves 2.

Zucchini, Eggplant, and Pepper Stew

This stew is a beautiful combination of vegetables that are at their best in late summer when soups and stews begin to call the appetite. If you have a garden of your own, this is a great way to make use of all that zucchini and eggplant that's coming in.

- 1 eggplant, cut into 1-inch cubes
- ¼ cup coconut oil
- 1 cup chopped onion
- 5 cloves garlic, chopped
- ½ cup cooked quinoa or brown rice
- 1 zucchini, cut into large chunks
- 1 large red bell pepper, chopped

- 3 fresh tomatoes, diced
- 1½ cups water
- 1 cup vegetable stock
- ½ teaspoon salt
- ¼ teaspoon crushed red pepper flakes
- ¼ cup chopped fresh basil
- ¼ cup chopped fresh parsley
- 1 sprig fresh rosemary, chopped

---

1. Place the eggplant cubes on a plate lined with paper towels and sprinkle with salt. Allow the eggplant to sweat for 15 minutes to draw out excess water. Rinse the eggplant and pat very dry.

2. Heat the coconut oil in a large pot over medium-high heat. Sauté the eggplant for 2 minutes on each side, or until lightly browned. Stir in the onion and sauté until transparent. Stir in the garlic and sauté for 2–3 more minutes.

3. Add the quinoa, zucchini, bell pepper, tomatoes, water, stock, salt, and red pepper flakes, and stir well. Cook just until the mixture reaches a low boil; then reduce the heat to medium-low and simmer for 45 minutes, or until the vegetables are tender.

4. Remove from the heat, and stir in the basil, parsley, and rosemary before serving.

Serves 6.

Tempeh Fajita Filling

Tempeh makes a great substitute for meat fillings in fajitas, tacos, and other Mexican fare. It absorbs the spicy flavors of Mexican food even better than meat and is adaptable to almost any recipe you may already have.

- 2 tablespoons coconut oil
- 1 (8-ounce) package tempeh, broken into pieces
- 2 tablespoons soy sauce
- 1 tablespoon freshly squeezed lime juice
- 1½ cups chopped green bell pepper
- ½ cup sliced fresh button mushrooms
- ½ cup chopped frozen spinach
- 1 tablespoon chopped green chili peppers
- 1 tablespoon chopped fresh cilantro
- 1 tablespoon dried minced onion

1. Heat the coconut oil in a large skillet over medium heat. Add the tempeh and stir in the soy sauce and lime juice. Sauté until the tempeh is browned, about 5 minutes.

2. Stir in the bell pepper, mushrooms, spinach, green chili peppers, cilantro, and dried onion. Increase the heat to medium-high and cook, stirring occasionally, for about 15 minutes, or until most of the liquid has evaporated.

Serves 4.

Vegetable Masala

Masala is a wonderfully fragrant and comforting dish that just draws people to the table. You can find garam masala in international markets or the spice section of larger grocery stores. This dish will taste even better the next day.

- 2 large potatoes, peeled and cubed
- 1 carrot, chopped
- 1 cup chopped fresh green beans
- ½ cup frozen peas, thawed
- 1 teaspoon salt
- ½ teaspoon ground turmeric
- 1 quart cold water
- 1 tablespoon coconut oil
- 1 teaspoon mustard seed

- 1 teaspoon ground cumin
- 1 large onion, finely chopped
- 2 large ripe tomatoes, cored and chopped
- 1 teaspoon garam masala
- ½ teaspoon ground ginger
- ½ teaspoon garlic powder
- ½ teaspoon chili powder
- 1 sprig cilantro leaves, for garnish

1. In a large microwave-safe dish, combine the potatoes, carrot, green beans, peas, salt, turmeric, and cold water. Cook for 8 minutes on high.

2. Heat the coconut oil in a large skillet over medium heat. Add the mustard seed and cumin, and heat just until the seeds start to pop. Add the onion and cook for about 3 minutes, or until transparent.

3. Stir in the tomatoes, garam masala, ginger, garlic powder, and chili powder, and cook for 3 minutes. Add the cooked vegetables to the mixture and sauté for 1 minute.

4. Garnish with cilantro leaves and serve.

Serves 4.

Vegan Shepherd's Pie

Shepherd's pie is one of those classic dishes that everyone in the family loves, from the youngest to the oldest. This version is meatless but every bit as delicious as the traditional preparation. This freezes very well; make two and pop one in the freezer for another time.

- 2 cups vegetable stock, divided
- 1 teaspoon yeast extract spread
- ½ cup dry lentils
- ¼ cup uncooked pearl barley
- 1 large carrot, diced
- ½ large yellow onion, finely chopped
- ½ cup walnuts, coarsely chopped
- 3 medium potatoes, chopped
- 1 teaspoon cornstarch
- ½ teaspoon water
- ½ teaspoon salt
- ¼ teaspoon freshly ground black pepper

1. Preheat oven to 350 degrees F.

2. In a large stockpot over medium-low heat, combine 1¼ cups of the vegetable stock, the yeast extract, lentils, and barley. Cook for 30 minutes, stirring occasionally.

3. Meanwhile, in a medium saucepan over medium-high heat, combine the remaining ¾ cup stock, carrot, onion, and walnuts. Simmer until the vegetables are tender, about 15 minutes.

4. While the vegetables cook, bring a large pot of salted water to a boil. Add the potatoes and cook until tender, about 15 minutes. Drain and mash.

5. Whisk the cornstarch and ½ teaspoon water with a fork until smooth, and stir into the carrot mixture. Simmer until thickened.

6. Add the carrot mixture to the lentils, and season with the salt and pepper. Pour the mixture into a 2-quart casserole dish. Spoon the mashed potatoes over the top, forming a crust, and bake until lightly browned, about 30 minutes.

Serves 6.

Lentil and Vegetable Casserole

This recipe is a great one to make when the air is cool and you want something to pop into the oven that will fill the house with a wonderful fragrance. You can use either red or yellow lentils for this recipe.

- ½ cup uncooked brown rice
- 2½ cups water, divided
- 1 cup red or yellow lentils
- 1 teaspoon coconut oil
- 1 small onion, chopped
- 3 cloves garlic, minced
- 1 medium fresh tomato, chopped
- ½ cup chopped celery
- ½ cup chopped carrots
- ½ cup chopped zucchini
- 1 (8-ounce) can tomato sauce
- 1 teaspoon dried basil
- 1 teaspoon dried oregano
- 1 teaspoon ground cumin
- ½ teaspoon salt
- ¼ teaspoon freshly ground black pepper

1. Place the brown rice and 1 cup of water in a large pot over high heat and bring to a boil. Cover, reduce the heat to low, and simmer for 20 minutes.

2. Place the lentils in another large pot with 1½ cups of water and bring to a boil. Cook for 15 minutes, or until the lentils are tender.

3. Preheat oven to 350 degrees F.

4. Heat the coconut oil in a large skillet over medium-high heat. Stir in the onion and garlic. Add the tomato, celery, carrots, zucchini, and half of the tomato sauce. Season with half the basil, half the oregano, half the cumin, and the salt and pepper. Cook until the vegetables are tender, about 15 minutes.

5. Mix the rice, lentils, and vegetables together in a large casserole dish, and pour the remaining half of the tomato sauce over the top. Season with the remaining basil, oregano, and cumin, and bake for 30 minutes, or until bubbly.

Serves 6.

Savory Vegan Nut Roast

This dish is similar to a nice meatloaf and makes a great plant-based entrée that will please even picky eaters. This is also excellent as a sandwich or lettuce wrap filling. The nut loaf will freeze quite nicely if you'd like to make extra batches for future meals.

- Coconut oil, for greasing pan
- 2 medium onions, chopped
- ½ cup chopped celery
- 1 tablespoon cold water
- 3 cups whole grain bread crumbs
- 2½ cups coconut milk

- ¾ cup walnuts
- ¾ cup pecan or sunflower meal
- 1 teaspoon dried basil
- 1 teaspoon dried oregano
- ½ teaspoon salt
- ¼ teaspoon freshly ground black pepper

1. Preheat the oven to 350 degrees F, and lightly grease a loaf pan with coconut oil.

2. In a medium skillet over medium-high heat, simmer the onion and celery with the cold water until cooked through, about 5 minutes.

3. Transfer the mixture to a large bowl, and add the bread crumbs, coconut milk, walnuts, pecan meal, basil, oregano, salt, and pepper. Stir until well blended.

4. Place the mixture into the prepared loaf pan. Bake for 60 minutes, or until the loaf is cooked through.

Serves 4.

Tofu Turkey Roast

This recipe will make an excellent substitute for a traditional roasted turkey breast. The tofu absorbs all of the traditional herbs and has a texture that is firm enough to stand in for the meat. The delectable orange glaze takes it to another level. Serve it for dinner one night, and make sandwiches with it the next day. Note that the tofu needs to chill for several hours before proceeding with the recipe.

- 5 (1-pound) packages extra-firm tofu, crumbled
- 2 tablespoons sesame oil, plus additional for greasing the pan
- 1 red onion, finely diced
- 1⅓ cups diced celery
- 1 cup chopped mushrooms
- 2 cloves garlic, minced
- 2 teaspoons dried sage
- 2 teaspoons dried thyme
- 1½ teaspoons dried rosemary
- ½ cup tamari, divided
- Salt and freshly ground black pepper to taste
- 3 cups vegan herb stuffing
- ½ cup coconut oil
- 5 tablespoons orange juice
- 2 tablespoons red miso paste
- 1 teaspoon honey mustard
- ½ teaspoon orange zest
- 3 sprigs fresh rosemary

1. Line a large colander with cheesecloth or several layers of paper towel. Place the crumbled tofu in the colander. Place another piece of cheesecloth over the top of the tofu. Place the colander over a large bowl. Place a heavy plate with cans or other weights on top of the tofu. Refrigerate for 2–3 hours.

2. In a large skillet over medium-high heat, heat the sesame oil. Add the onion, celery, and mushrooms, and sauté until tender. Add the garlic, sage, thyme, rosemary, and ¼ cup of tamari. Season with the salt and pepper, and sauté for 5 minutes. Add the herb stuffing and mix well. Remove from the heat and set aside.

3. Preheat oven to 400 degrees F. Grease a baking sheet with just a bit of sesame oil.

4. In a small bowl, combine the remaining ¼ cup tamari, coconut oil, orange juice, miso, honey mustard, and orange zest, and whisk until well blended.

5. Remove the weight from the tofu. Scoop out just enough of the tofu to leave a 1-inch tofu lining inside the colander. Place the scooped-out tofu in a separate bowl.

6. Brush the tofu lining with a small amount of the seasoning sauce. Spoon the vegetable stuffing into the center of the tofu shell.

7. Place the reserved tofu on top of the stuffing and press down firmly. Gently flip the colander over to place the stuffed tofu onto the prepared baking sheet. Gently mold the sides of the tofu turkey to form an oval shape.

8. Brush the tofu turkey with half of the seasoning sauce. Top with the rosemary sprigs and cover the tofu with foil.

9. Bake for 1 hour. After 1 hour, remove the foil. Baste the tofu turkey with the remaining seasoning sauce. Return the tofu turkey to the oven and bake for 1 more hour, or until golden brown.

Serves 8-10.

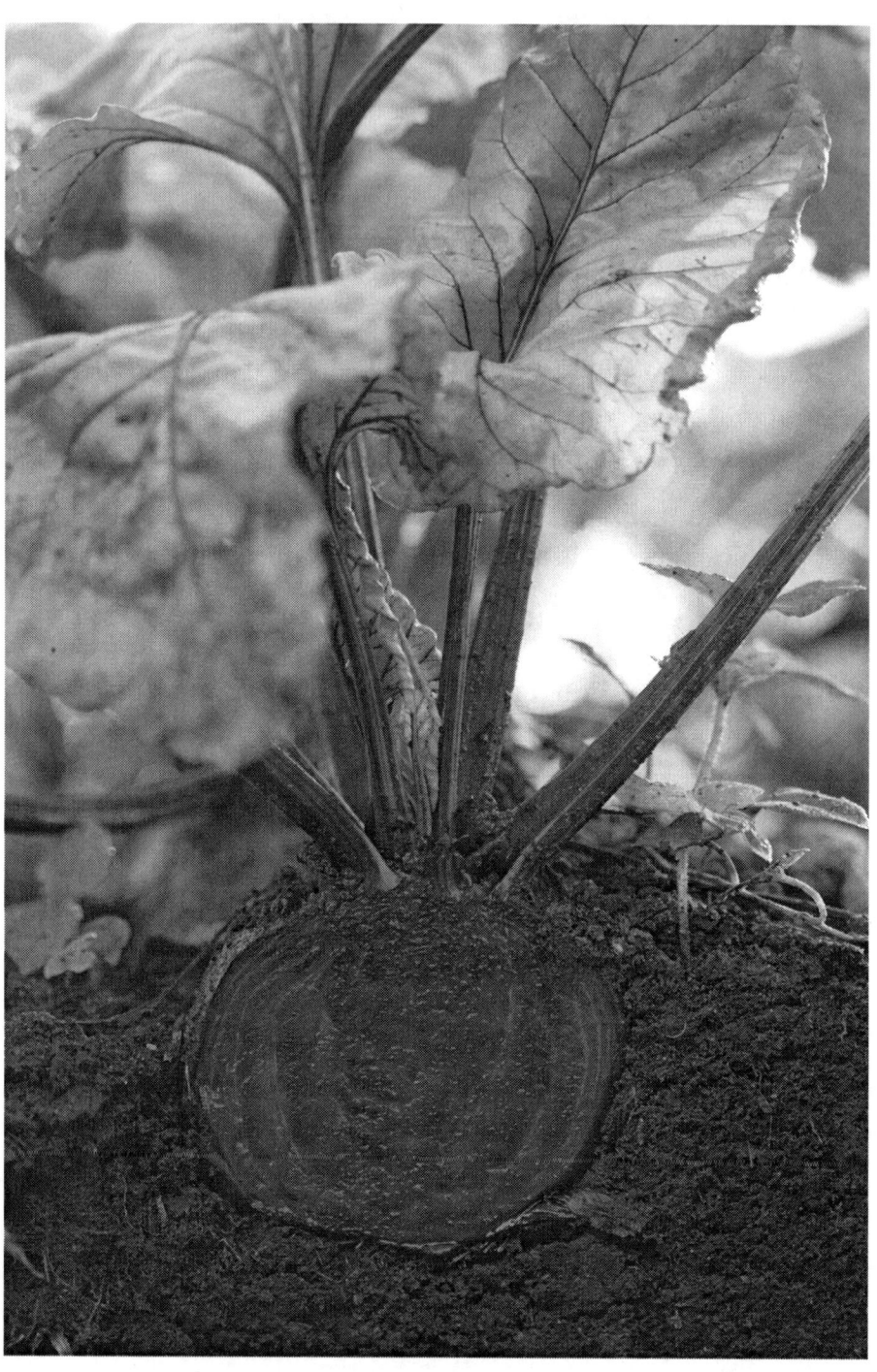

Beets have been shown to lower blood pressure and increase athletic performance.

10

CHINA STUDY DIET SIDE DISHES

Roasted Asparagus and Mushrooms

Simple and delicious. A small ingredient list means less room for error and less time needed to put together a side dish that's perfect on a busy night. You can use any type of fresh mushroom for this recipe.

- 1 pound fresh asparagus, tough bottoms trimmed
- 1 cup sliced fresh mushrooms
- 2 cloves garlic
- ½ teaspoon smoked paprika
- ½ teaspoon salt
- ¼ teaspoon freshly ground black pepper
- 1 teaspoon coconut oil

1. Preheat oven to 375 degrees F. Line a baking sheet with aluminum foil.

2. In a large ziplock bag, combine the asparagus, mushrooms, garlic, paprika, salt, pepper, and coconut oil. Seal and knead the bag to coat the vegetables well.

3. Spread the vegetables on the baking sheet. Bake for about 20 minutes, or until the asparagus is tender but not dry.

Serves 4.

Oven-Baked Potato Medley

This side dish looks and tastes beautiful. Cooked in coconut oil, this red-and-sweet-potato mixture caramelizes beautifully, enhancing the natural sweetness of the tubers. Wonderful served alongside steamed or roasted veggies.

- 2 cups red potatoes, cut into bite-sized chunks
- 2 cups sweet potatoes (skin on), cut into bite-sized chunks
- ½ teaspoon salt
- ½ teaspoon freshly ground black pepper
- 2 tablespoons coconut oil
- 1 teaspoon fresh dill leaves

1. Preheat oven to 425 degrees F.

2. In a glass baking dish, combine the red potatoes, sweet potatoes, salt, pepper, and coconut oil. Stir until all the potatoes are well coated. Bake until the potatoes are tender, about 45 minutes.

3. Stir in the dill, and let sit for 5 minutes before serving.

Serves 4.

Savory Quinoa

Everyone needs comfort food, but that doesn't mean it can't be as healthful as it is good. This dish is a great substitute for rice but packs a lot more protein and omega-3 fatty acids. Serve alongside a salad or stir into vegetable soups to make them more hearty.

- 2 cups uncooked quinoa
- 4 cups water
- Pinch of salt
- 2 medium zucchini, chopped
- 1 medium onion, finely chopped
- 4 cloves garlic
- 1 cup of coconut milk
- Freshly ground black pepper to taste

1. Rinse the quinoa and drain well.

2. Bring the quinoa, water, and a pinch of salt to a boil in a medium pot over medium-high heat. Reduce the heat to medium-low and simmer for 20–30 minutes, or until the quinoa begins to look translucent. Do not stir or the quinoa will not be fluffy.

3. Meanwhile, combine the zucchini, onion, garlic, and coconut milk in a food processor or blender, and blend until very smooth and creamy. Season with the salt and pepper.

4. In a medium saucepan over medium-high heat, bring the puree to a simmer and let it cook, stirring occasionally, for about 10 minutes or until soft.

5. Serve the quinoa with the puree poured over it, or stir together before serving.

Serves 4.

Oven-Roasted Vegetable Medley

There is a lot of variety in this dish, but the flavors blend together gracefully. The natural flavors of the vegetables are enhanced by the roasting alone, allowing you to savor them for what they are — pure, fresh goodness.

- 1 cup fresh broccoli florets, broken into pieces
- 1 cup fresh cauliflower florets, broken into pieces
- 1 cup baby carrots
- ½ medium onion, chopped
- 4 cloves garlic, crushed
- 2 tablespoons coconut oil
- 2 tablespoons chopped fresh parsley
- ½ teaspoon salt
- ¼ teaspoon freshly ground black pepper

1. Preheat oven to 425 degrees F.

2. Combine all of the ingredients in a large bowl, and toss until the vegetables are well coated with the coconut oil and seasonings.

3. Spread in a single layer in a large baking dish. Bake for about 45 minutes, or until the vegetables are tender.

Serves 4.

Fried Coconut Bananas

Don't be fooled, this isn't candy, but it is a great way to get the kids excited about dinner. This dish is excellent with almost any entrée but would be especially good with the Tofu Turkey Roast presented earlier in the book. Choose bananas that are ripe but still firm; they'll hold their shape best.

- 3 bananas, sliced at an angle
- ½ cup shredded coconut
- ¼ cup coconut oil

1. Roll the sliced bananas in the shredded coconut until well covered.

2. Melt the coconut oil in a large skillet over medium heat, and sauté the bananas until the coconut is browned.

Serves 4.

Vegan Potatoes au Gratin

Using vegan soy cheese in this recipe allows you to create a dish that is every bit as satisfying and creamy as the traditional version. This is a real hit with children and guests who may not know how delicious vegan food can be.

- 6 large potatoes, peeled and cubed
- 2 quarts water
- 1¼ cups vegetable stock, divided
- 2 tablespoons arrowroot powder
- 1 teaspoon salt

- ½ teaspoon freshly ground black pepper
- ¼ teaspoon dry mustard
- ¼ teaspoon ground nutmeg
- 2 cups soy milk
- 1½ cups shredded cheddar-flavored soy cheese, divided
- 1 cup fresh bread crumbs
- 1 tablespoon paprika

1. Preheat oven to 350 degrees F.

2. In a large pot, bring the water and some salt to a boil. Add the potatoes and cook until tender, about 15 minutes. Drain and place in a 9 x 13–inch baking dish.

3. Meanwhile, in a small saucepan over high heat, bring 2 tablespoons of the vegetable stock to a boil. Reduce the heat to low, and whisk in the arrowroot powder, salt, pepper, dry mustard, and nutmeg. Gradually add the soy milk, whisking constantly until thickened. Stir in half of the soy cheese. Whisk until the cheese is melted. Pour the sauce over the potatoes.

4. In a small bowl, mix the remaining 1 cup plus 2 tablespoons of vegetable stock and the bread crumbs. Spread evenly over the potatoes. Top with the remaining soy cheese and sprinkle with the paprika.

5. Bake the gratin for 20 minutes, or until golden.

Serves 8.

Veggie-Packed Couscous

This side dish is loaded with vegetables and layer upon layer of flavor. This is a wonderful dish to have as a side, but it's hearty enough for an entrée as well. Experiment with different varieties of vegetables for each season.

- 1 medium onion, julienned
- 3 cups vegetable stock
- 2 carrots, peeled and sliced into strips
- 2 turnips, peeled and sliced into strips
- 1 sweet potato, peeled and sliced into strips
- 1 orange bell pepper, peeled and sliced into strips
- 1 (15-ounce) can garbanzo beans, rinsed and drained
- 1 (12-ounce) can tomato sauce
- ¼ teaspoon ground cinnamon
- ½ teaspoon ground turmeric
- Pinch of saffron
- Pinch of curry powder
- 2½ cups water
- 2 cups uncooked couscous

1. In a large saucepan over medium heat, sauté the onion until it's browned. Add the vegetable stock and bring to a boil.

2. Once the stock is boiling, add the carrots, turnips, and sweet potato to the pan. Simmer for 15–20 minutes. Reduce the heat to medium-low, add the bell pepper, and continue simmering for 20 minutes.

3. Stir in the beans, tomato sauce, cinnamon, turmeric, saffron, and curry powder. Continue cooking until the sauce is heated through.

4. Meanwhile, in a medium pot over medium-high heat, bring the water to a boil. Add the couscous, cover, remove from the heat, and let sit for 5 minutes. Fluff the couscous with a fork and serve with the vegetable mixture over the top.

Serves 6.

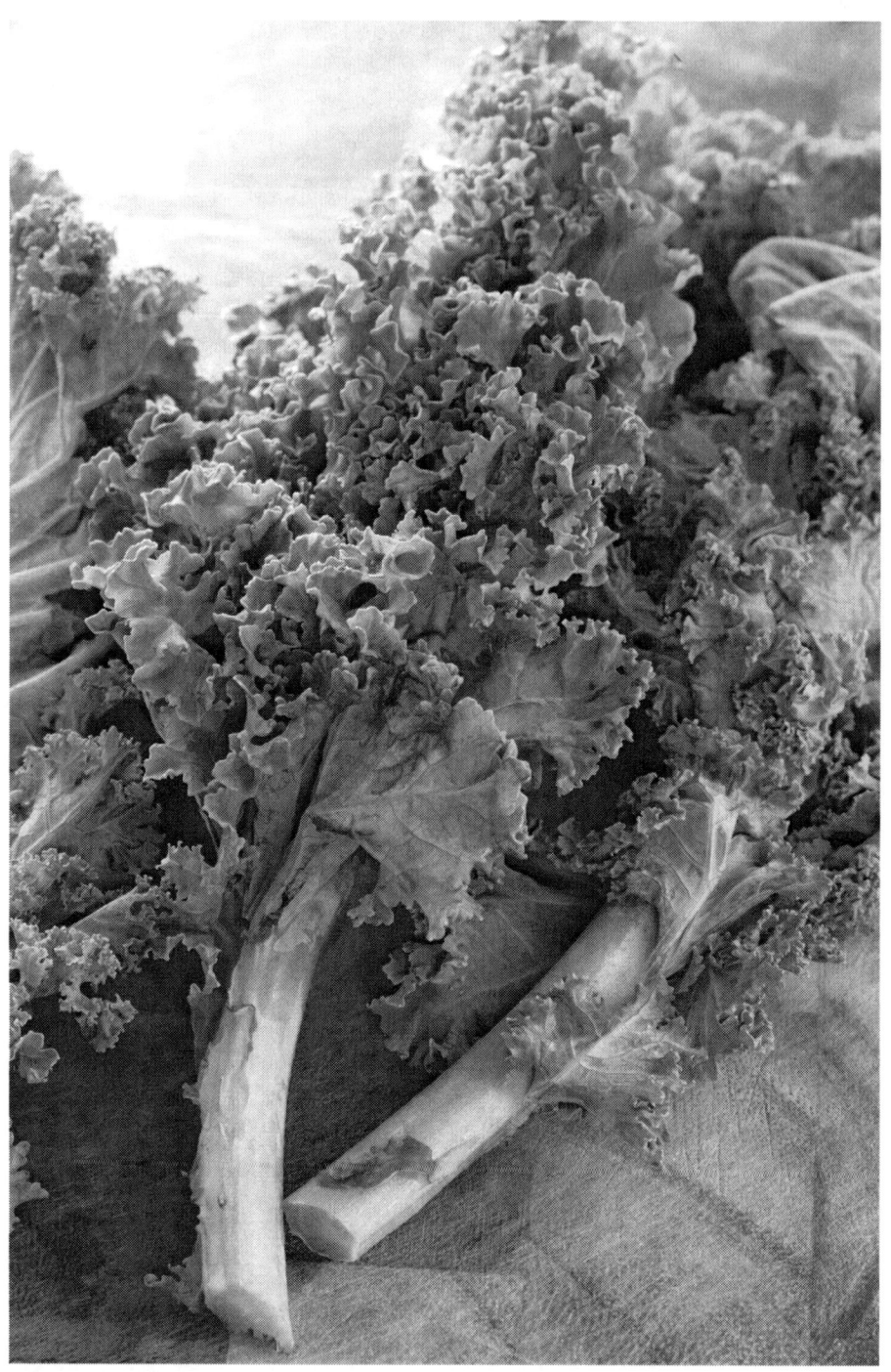
Kale is one of the dark leafy greens that is at its best when hit with a touch of frost, making it an excellent choice in winter, when other greens are imported or unavailable.

Brussels with a Kick

With just enough spice to clear the airways, these tiny little cabbages will definitely be remembered. The spice can be toned down if needed, but you won't sacrifice any of the flavor.

- ½ pound brussels sprouts, ends trimmed
- 2 tablespoons plus 1 teaspoon coconut oil
- ¼ teaspoon crushed red pepper flakes
- ¼ teaspoon cayenne pepper
- 1 tablespoon liquid smoke seasoning, divided
- 1 tablespoon capers, roughly chopped
- 1 tablespoon balsamic vinegar

1. Prepare the brussels sprouts by removing the outer leaves and then washing them in a colander. Slice them in half lengthwise.

2. Heat a large skillet over medium-high heat and melt the coconut oil. Add the red pepper flakes, cayenne, and about ¼ teaspoon of the liquid smoke. Stir well.

3. Place the brussels sprouts cut side down in the pan and allow them to cook, untouched, for about 5 minutes, or until nicely browned. Stir the sprouts and continue cooking until each one is slightly charred and tender.

4. Add the remaining ¾ teaspoon liquid smoke, capers, and balsamic vinegar, and stir once. Serve immediately.

Serves 4.

Noodles with Green Beans

As simple as it sounds, kids will eat just about anything if it is mixed with noodles, so this is a great dish to serve younger members of the family.

- 1 pound green beans, trimmed and halved
- 1 pound whole grain penne pasta
- 1 teaspoon coconut oil
- 1 medium onion, chopped
- ½ teaspoon crushed garlic
- 1 teaspoon soy sauce
- ¼ teaspoon freshly ground black pepper

1. In a medium pot over medium-high heat, cook the green beans in boiling water until tender. Drain well.

2. Meanwhile, cook the pasta in boiling salted water until al dente. Drain and set aside.

3. Melt the coconut oil in a large skillet over medium heat, and add the onion and garlic. Sauté for 5 minutes. Add the green beans and sauté for 5–7 minutes, or until crisp but slightly tender.

4. Add the soy sauce and toss well. Stir in the pasta and pepper, and serve immediately.

Serves 4.

Sautéed Kale with Garlic

Kale goes beautifully with fresh garlic and is loaded with iron and fiber. It will sauté very quickly and it makes a nice change from spinach or other greens. You can save time by buying the kale already trimmed of its tough ribs.

- 1 tablespoon coconut oil
- 1 large bunch fresh kale, ribs removed, washed and drained
- 3 cloves garlic, crushed
- ½ teaspoon salt
- ¼ teaspoon freshly ground black pepper

1. In a large skillet over medium-high heat, melt the coconut oil. Toss in the kale by the handful and allow it to wilt for a minute to accommodate all of the kale. Add the garlic, salt, and pepper, and sauté, stirring frequently, for 5 minutes.

Serves 4.

Tangy Sweet Baked Beans

Baked beans made from scratch are so superior to what you can buy in the store. Cooking with dried beans does take time, but it's incredibly economical, easy to do, and very satisfying in the end. This recipe uses navy beans, but you could also substitute great northern if you like.

- 1 pound dry navy beans
- 6 cups water
- 2 tablespoons coconut oil
- 2 cups chopped sweet onion
- 1 clove garlic, minced
- 4 (8-ounce) cans tomato sauce
- ¼ cup pure maple syrup
- ¼ cup molasses
- 2 tablespoons apple cider vinegar
- 3 bay leaves
- 1 teaspoon dry mustard
- ¼ teaspoon freshly ground black pepper
- ¼ teaspoon ground nutmeg
- ¼ teaspoon ground cinnamon

1. Place the navy beans and water in a large stockpot, and bring to a boil. Reduce the heat to medium-low and continue cooking for 1 hour, stirring occasionally, until the beans are tender. Drain the beans and discard any liquid. Pour the beans into a large baking dish.

2. Preheat oven to 300 degrees F.

3. In a medium skillet over medium-high heat, melt the coconut oil and stir in the onions. Cook for 3 minutes, or until tender. Add the garlic and sauté until golden brown. Stir the onion mixture into the beans.

4. In a large bowl, stir together the tomato sauce, maple syrup, molasses, vinegar, bay leaves, dry mustard, pepper, nutmeg, and cinnamon until well blended. Then stir into the beans, mixing well.

5. Cover the baking dish and bake for 3½ hours, stirring frequently and adding water as needed to keep the beans moist. Uncover and continue baking for 30 more minutes.

Serves 10.

Asian-Style Mustard Greens

Mustard greens are absolutely delicious and loaded with iron, folate, and other nutrients. They're also an excellent source of fiber. In Southern American cooking, they're often cooked down to nothing, but this Asian-influenced recipe leaves them flavorful and fresh.

- 2 tablespoons sesame seeds
- 1 teaspoon coconut oil
- 6 cups chopped fresh mustard greens

- ¼ cup water
- 2 teaspoons minced garlic
- 1 tablespoon soy sauce
- 2 teaspoons mirin
- 1 teaspoon honey

1. Heat a large skillet over medium heat and add the sesame seeds. Toast, stirring constantly, until the seeds are golden brown and popping, about 1–2 minutes. Remove the sesame seeds immediately to a small bowl to cool.

2. Melt the coconut oil in the hot skillet, and then add the mustard greens and water. Stir the mustard greens until they are wilted and reduced in size by about half. Stir in the garlic, soy sauce, mirin, and honey.

3. Bring the mixture to a boil, stirring constantly, and then reduce the heat to low and cover. Simmer for 10–15 minutes, or until the greens are tender.

4. Remove the greens from the skillet with a slotted spoon, increase the heat to high, and simmer the liquid until reduced by half. Return the greens to the pan and stir until heated through.

5. Sprinkle with the sesame seeds before serving.

Serves 4.

Glazed Carrots

Carrots are beautifully sweet on their own, but when glazed and allowed to develop their sweetness, they're almost better than candy. This side dish would go beautifully with a heaping plate of greens or a baked potato.

- 6 large carrots, quartered
- 2 cloves garlic, minced
- 3 tablespoons light soy sauce
- 3 tablespoons rice vinegar
- 4 teaspoons honey
- 2 teaspoons coconut oil
- 2 teaspoons minced fresh ginger
- ¼ teaspoon Chinese five-spice powder

1. Fill a large pot with cold water and bring to a boil over high heat. Add the carrots and cook for 5 minutes. Drain and rinse with cold water, and then pat dry.

2. In a large, nonmetallic bowl or dish, combine the remaining ingredients, stirring well. Add the carrots, toss to coat, and let marinate for 30 minutes.

3. Heat a large skillet over medium-high heat, and cook the carrots in a single layer for about 5 minutes on each side, or until caramelized and glossy. Serve hot.

Serves 6.

Curried Sweet Potatoes

Sweet potatoes are loaded with iron, fiber, and more protein than usually found in a plant-based food. They also contain less starch than white potatoes. This method of preparing them is simple, but the flavors are different enough to make the dish quite special.

- 4 medium sweet potatoes, scrubbed
- 4 teaspoons coconut oil, melted
- 1 teaspoon honey
- 1 teaspoon mild curry powder
- ½ teaspoon paprika
- ½ teaspoon salt
- ¼ teaspoon freshly ground black pepper

1. Preheat oven to 400 degrees F.

2. Place the potatoes on a baking sheet, prick each one several times with a fork, and bake for 50–60 minutes, or until quite tender. Allow the potatoes to cool enough to be handled, but still very warm.

3. Slice just the top ¼ inch or so lengthwise from each potato, and gently scoop the flesh into a medium glass bowl, reserving the skins. Mash the flesh with a fork until chunky but somewhat smooth.

4. In a small bowl, combine the melted coconut oil, honey, curry powder, paprika, salt, and pepper, and stir until well combined.

5. Pour into the sweet potato flesh, and stir well with a fork to combine. Spoon back into the potato skins, leaving the filling fluffy.

Serves 4.

Spinach with Mushrooms and Peppers

Spinach is one of the fastest-cooking greens, which makes it perfect for a quick side dish on a busy night. In this recipe, the crunch and sweetness of red peppers and the woody flavor of mushrooms enhance the spinach's delicate flavor.

- 1 teaspoon coconut oil
- 1 clove garlic, minced
- ½ medium red bell pepper, diced
- ½ small sweet onion, diced
- 1 pound fresh spinach leaves, rinsed and well drained
- ½ pound sliced fresh mushrooms
- ½ teaspoon salt
- ¼ teaspoon freshly ground black pepper

1. In a large skillet over medium-high heat, melt the coconut oil. Once hot, add the garlic, bell pepper, and onion, and sauté for 5 minutes, stirring frequently. Add the spinach, mushrooms, salt, and pepper, stirring well to combine. Sauté for 5 more minutes, or just until the spinach is wilted and the mushrooms are slightly golden.

Serves 4.

11

CHINA STUDY DIET DESSERTS

Strawberry-Pineapple Compote over Homemade Coconut Ice Cream

This dessert is a great one to serve to guests. It looks like it's breaking the rules, but this dessert is 100 percent vegan and absolutely delicious.

For the compote:
- 1 cup sliced fresh strawberries
- 1 cup chopped fresh pineapple
- 2 tablespoons pure maple syrup
- 1 cinnamon stick

- ½ teaspoon crushed red pepper flakes
- ¼ teaspoon lime zest

For the ice cream:
- 1 (15-ounce) can cream of coconut
- 1½ cups refrigerated coconut milk (not canned)

Make the compote:

1. Combine the strawberries and pineapple in a skillet over medium-low heat. Sauté until the pineapple is lightly browned.

2. Add the maple syrup, cinnamon stick, and red pepper flakes, and lightly simmer until the fruit has caramelized, about 2–3 minutes.

3. Remove the cinnamon stick and add the lime zest. Give the compote one last stir.

4. Let cool to room temperature.

Make the ice cream:

5. Add all of the ingredients to an ice-cream maker, and process according to the manufacturer's instructions.

6. To serve, scoop the ice cream into bowls and top with the compote.

Serves 4.

Sweet Berry, No Dairy Parfait

When you are really in dire need of a creamy treat, you can whip this up in minutes and indulge your cravings without worrying about what it's doing to your health. This is a real hit with the kids as well. You can make the granola in large batches and store in an airtight container for up to 3 weeks.

For the granola:
- ½ cup old-fashioned oats
- ½ cup chopped almonds or other hard nut
- ¼ cup pure maple syrup

For the parfait:
- 3 cups vegan yogurt, preferably coconut or almond
- ½ cup sliced fresh strawberries
- ½ cup fresh blueberries

Make the granola:

1. Line a baking sheet with parchment paper.

2. In a medium bowl, stir together the oats and almonds, and then add the maple syrup. Fold the ingredients together until everything is well coated. The mixture will be slightly hard to work with and should be very clumpy.

3. Break granola crumbles evenly over the parchment paper, spreading them out. Let the crumbles sit in the refrigerator for 5 minutes.

Make the parfait:

4. Lightly mix the yogurt and berries together.

5. To serve, spoon the parfait into bowls and top with the granola.

Serves 4.

Coconut-Coated Fruit Balls

This serves as a quick fix for a midday snack or a midnight sweet tooth. The balls are packed with good-for-you ingredients, are naturally sweet, and are also great for when you need a real energy boost. The fruit balls will keep well in an airtight container for up to a week.

- 1 cup sliced almonds, broken into pieces
- 1 cup dried apple rings with cinnamon
- 1 cup unsweetened raw coconut flakes
- 1 cup fresh soft dates
- ¾ cup dried cranberries

---

1. Lay a large piece of parchment paper on the countertop or on a cookie sheet.

2. Combine the almonds, dried apples, coconut flakes, and dates in a food processor, and pulse until they begin to bind together. Add the cranberries and pulse just a few times, allowing for chunks of cranberry to remain throughout the mixture.

3. Roll about 1½ tablespoons of the mixture in the palm of your hand to form a ball. Place the ball on the parchment paper. Repeat this process until the mixture is gone. Allow the balls to set for about 30 minutes before serving.

Makes about 20 fruit balls.

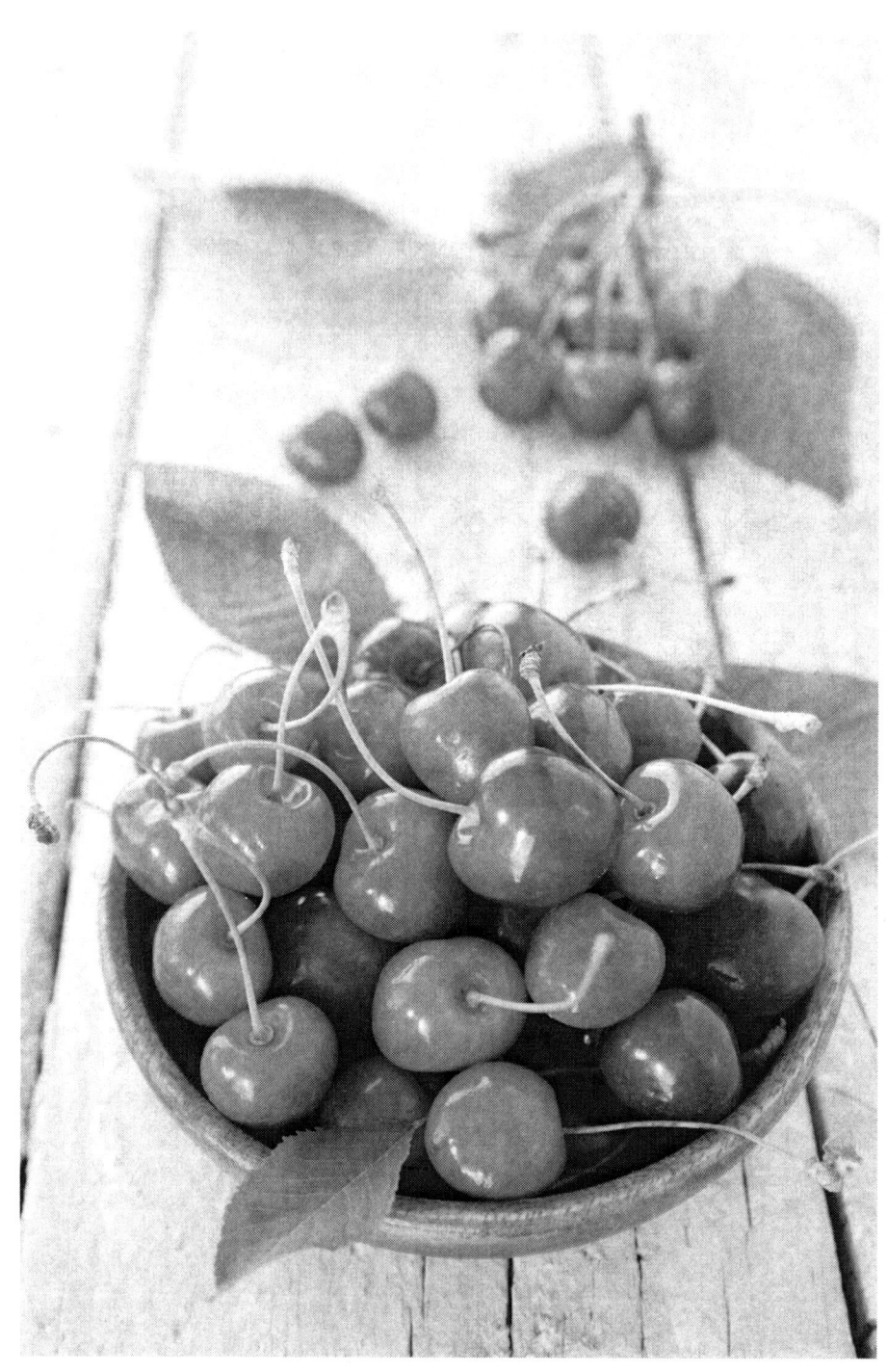

Sour cherries are higher in vitamin C than sweet cherries.

Bake-Less No Face Cookies

These cookies are not too sweet but sure to cure the craving if your sweet tooth starts making demands. They are also packed with plenty of plant-based protein and fiber, which are essential for disease prevention.

- ½ cup coconut milk
- ½ cup vegan butter
- 1 teaspoon pure vanilla extract
- 3½ cups quick oats
- ½ cup almond butter
- ¼ cup unsweetened cocoa powder

1. Combine the coconut milk, vegan butter, and vanilla in a small saucepan over medium heat, and stir occasionally until smooth and creamy, about 10 minutes.

2. Combine the oats, almond butter, and cocoa powder in a large bowl, and stir until well blended. Be careful not to leave any clumps of cocoa powder.

3. Pour the warm coconut milk mixture over the oat mixture and mix well. Using a tablespoon, scoop spoonfuls of dough onto waxed paper, and let cool for about 30 minutes. The cookies should be chewy but firm.

Makes about 2 dozen cookies.

Maple Candy

This tiny decadent dessert is satisfyingly sweet but doesn't contain processed sugars or animal products. With its melt-in-your-mouth fudgelike texture, moderation is the only thing you need to worry about.

- 2 cups pure maple syrup
- 1 cup chopped walnuts
- ¼ cup dried cranberries or other dried fruit

1. In a large saucepan, bring the maple syrup to a boil over medium-high heat, stirring occasionally. It is important that the syrup reaches a temperature of 235 degrees F (110 degrees C) on a candy thermometer.

2. When the temperature is reached, remove the pan from the heat and let the syrup cool for about 10 minutes, or until the temperature lowers to about 170 degrees F (80 degrees C). Do not stir at all during this time.

3. Once cooled, stir the syrup constantly with a spoon for about 5 minutes, or until it turns a milky caramel color. Immediately stir in the walnuts and cranberries.

4. Pour the candy mixture into molds and let stand until completely cooled. The candies can be stored for up to 1 month in an airtight container.

Makes 18–20 candies.

Coco-Nut Cookies

These quick and easy chocolate almond cookies are completely free of refined sugars, dairy, and eggs, so they're a worry-free go-to snack for those times when the kids want a sweet treat. These will keep well for about 1 week in an airtight container or for 3 months in the freezer.

- 2 cups all-purpose whole wheat flour
- ½ cup thinly chopped almonds, pulsed in a food processor until granular
- 1½ tablespoons unsweetened raw cocoa powder
- 1 teaspoon aluminum-free baking powder
- ½ teaspoon baking soda
- ¼ teaspoon salt
- ½ cup coconut oil, melted
- ½ cup pure maple syrup
- ½ cup water
- 1 teaspoon pure vanilla extract

---

1. Preheat oven to 350 degrees F. If you have a convection oven setting, it works well with this recipe.

2. In a medium bowl, combine the flour, almonds, cocoa powder, baking powder, baking soda, and salt.

3. In a separate bowl, whisk together the coconut oil, maple syrup, water, and vanilla.

4. Add the wet ingredients to the flour mixture. Using a spatula, fold the ingredients together until they are well blended and form a dough.

5. Shape each cookie by placing 1 tablespoon of the dough on a cookie sheet and flattening it with a spoon.

6. Bake for 8–10 minutes, checking the cookies often without opening the oven door. The bottoms and edges should be golden brown.

7. Transfer the cookies to a wire rack to cool completely.

Makes 24–30 cookies.

Strawberry-Rhubarb Custard Pie

This recipe is well worth the labor! Antioxidant-rich, and delightfully creamy, it makes for a great spring or summer pie. The superb vegan pie crust is versatile enough to adapt for any recipe and will quickly become a standby in your home baking. This makes enough for a double crust; so simply freeze half of the dough for another day, or make two pies.

For the crust:
- 2 cups whole wheat flour
- ⅔ cup coconut oil
- ⅓ cup water
- Pinch of salt

For the filling:
- 3 cups rhubarb cut into ¼-inch-thick slices
- 1 cup fresh strawberries, quartered
- 3 tablespoons flaxseed mixed with 9 tablespoons water

- 3 tablespoons pure maple syrup
- 3 tablespoons coconut milk
- 3 tablespoons all-purpose whole wheat flour
- ¼ teaspoon ground nutmeg
- 1 tablespoon vegan butter, cut into small pieces

For the jam:
- 1 cup fresh strawberries, pureed in a food processor
- 1 tablespoon pure maple syrup

Make the crust:

1. Preheat oven to 350 degrees F.

2. Stir together all of the crust ingredients thoroughly to form a dough ball. Cut the dough in half and reserve one half. Wrap the second half in freezer paper, and seal in a ziplock freezer bag for later use.

3. Press the dough into a 9-inch pie pan. Prebake the crust for 8 minutes, and then set aside. Leave the oven at 350 degrees F.

Make the filling:

4. In a large bowl, combine the rhubarb and strawberries, and transfer to the pie crust. Make sure the fruit is distributed evenly.

5. Whisk together the flaxseed-water mixture, maple syrup, coconut milk, flour, and nutmeg until well blended. Slowly pour the liquid into the pie until it fills the shell. Scatter the vegan butter pieces evenly over the top of the pie. Gently tap the pan and shake it gently to remove all of the air bubbles.

6. Place the pan on the center oven rack and bake for 1 hour, or until the filling is set, turning once halfway through baking. Cool on a wire rack.

Make the jam:

7. Whisk the pureed strawberries and the maple syrup gently until blended. Microwave until warm, about 1 minute. Brush a thin layer over the top of the filling. Refrigerate the pie until ready to serve..

Makes 1 (9-inch) pie.

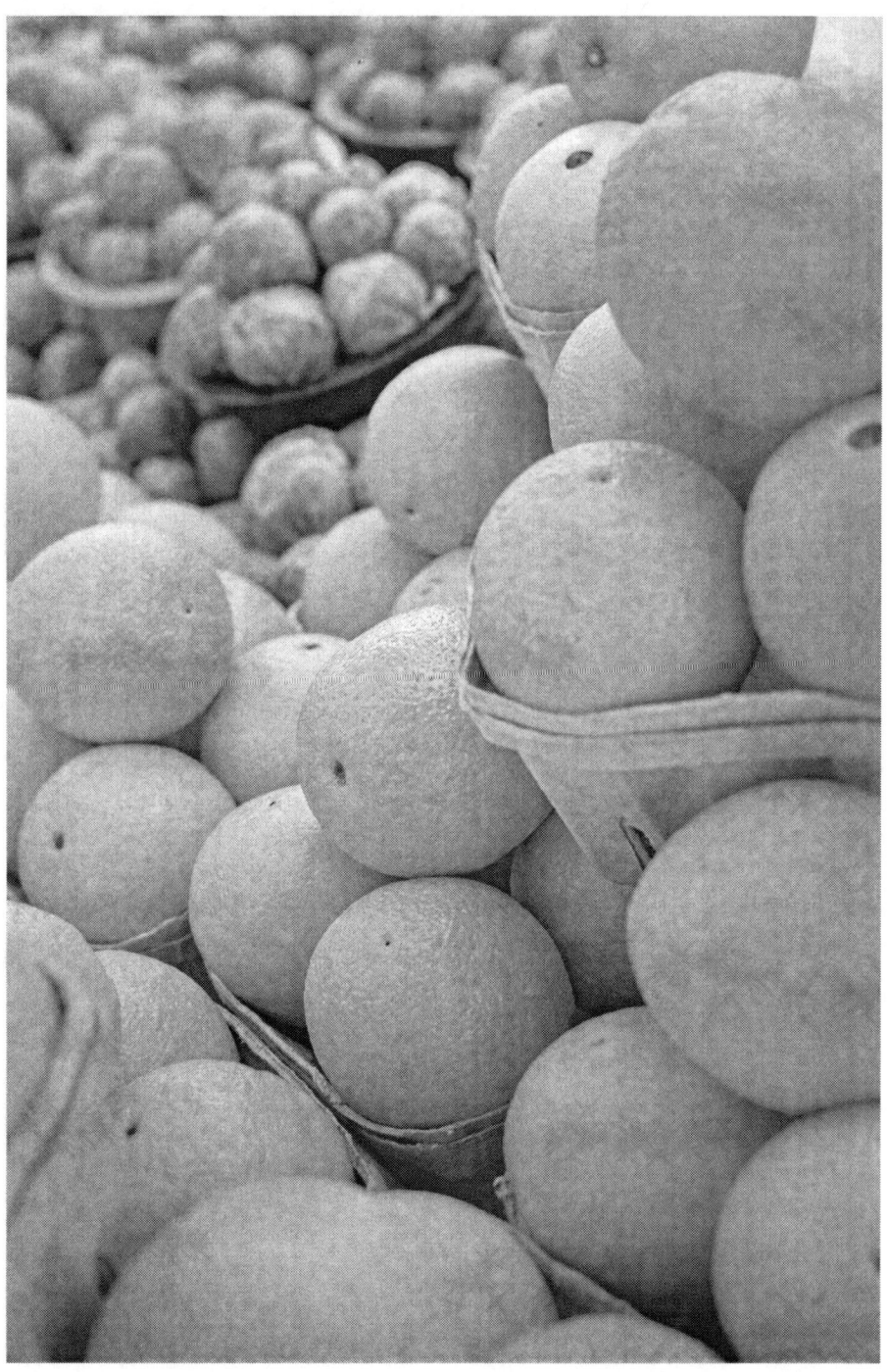

Although it's not as tasty as the flesh, the orange peel is edible and contains a high amount of vitamin C.

Vegan Coconut Rice Pudding

One of the hardest things to find 100 percent animal-, dairy-, egg-, and refined sugar-free is pudding. Here is a recipe that meets all those requirements and is also completely addictive. This rice pudding will bring back wonderful childhood memories.

- 3 cups cooked rice (cooked in coconut milk instead of water)
- 3 cups coconut milk
- 2 tablespoons pure maple syrup
- 2 tablespoons vegan butter
- 1 teaspoon pure vanilla extract
- Raisins (optional)
- Ground cinnamon (optional)

1. In a medium saucepan, bring the rice, coconut milk, maple syrup, vegan butter, and vanilla to a boil. Reduce to a simmer and stir occasionally for 25 minutes.

2. When most of the liquid is absorbed and the rice is creamy, add the raisins, if desired, and stir well to incorporate.

3. Spoon the rice pudding into bowls and sprinkle with cinnamon, if desired. Serve warm or cold.

Serves 4.

Berry Picnic Pie

This recipe is so simple that it will quickly become a family favorite. The pie would make a great picnic dessert or a treat to bring on a camping trip. It's loaded with protein and vitamin C, which makes it perfect to serve the kids.

For the crust:
- 1 cup raw whole almonds
- 1 cup raw walnuts
- 1 cup dates, pitted
- ½ teaspoon ground cardamom
- ½ teaspoon ground cinnamon

For the filling:
- 2½ cups frozen (thawed) blueberries

- 1 cup frozen (thawed) strawberries
- ⅓ cup dates, pitted
- ½ teaspoon ground cardamom
- ¼ teaspoon ground cinnamon

For garnish:
- 2 cups fresh blueberries, raspberries, or blackberries
- ½ kiwi, sliced
- Sliced almonds

Make the crust:

1. To make the crust, pulse the almonds and walnuts in a food processor for 2–3 minutes, or until the texture resembles a fine meal. Add the dates, cardamom, and cinnamon, and process for about 5 minutes, or until the mixture starts to bind together.

2. Press the crust mixture into a 9-inch pie pan by hand. Allow the crust to set in the refrigerator for 30 minutes, or until firm.

Make the filling:

3. To make the filling, add all of the ingredients to a clean food processor and process until pureed and smooth.

4. Fill the chilled crust and place the pie back into the refrigerator for 30–45 minutes, or until the filling has thickened and set slightly.

5. Lightly score the pie into eight slices before decorating. Garnish with the blueberries, kiwi, and almonds in any desired design, or just pile it all on and enjoy!

Makes 1 (9-inch) pie.

Banana-Blueberry Sorbet

This dessert is simple to make and delicately flavored. It's a wonderful dessert to serve company because it looks and tastes elegant, but it is so easy to prepare. Try using strawberries, raspberries, or blackberries, too. This recipe can easily be doubled or tripled to serve more.

• 2 bananas (the riper the better)	• 1 cup blueberries • ½ cup coconut milk

1. Add all of the ingredients to a food processor and process just until well blended.

2. Transfer the mixture to an ice-cream maker, and process according to the manufacturer's instructions.

Serves 2.

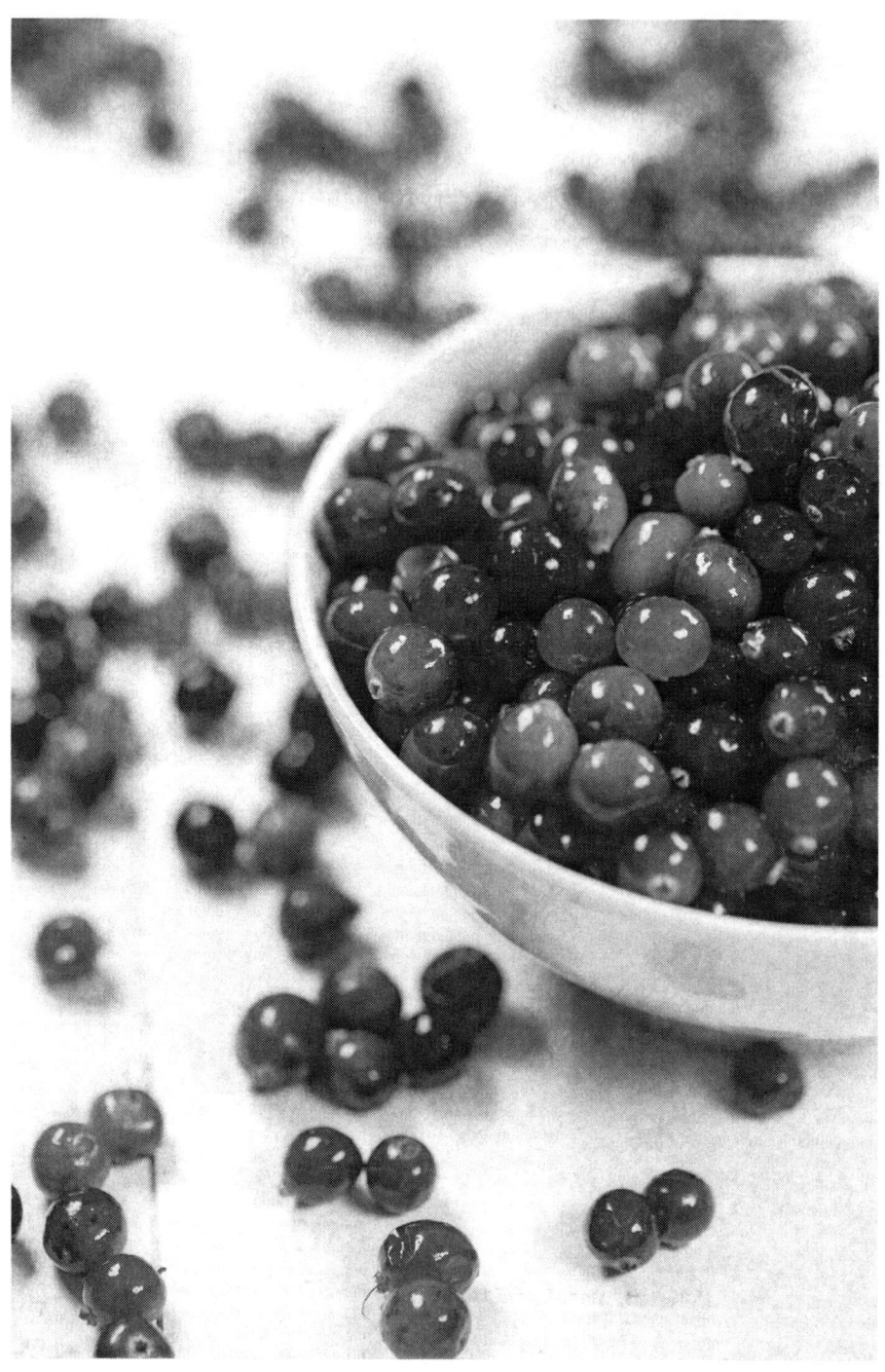

High in nutrients and antioxidants, raw cranberries are considered a "superfruit."

Delicious Fruit Pizza

This fruit dessert is so simple and so quick it can be whipped up in minutes. This recipe is great to use for cooking with children and helping them to see how delicious and fun healthful foods can be. Experiment with any fruits at the peak of freshness.

- 1 large whole wheat tortilla
- 1 teaspoon coconut oil
- Pure maple syrup
- Pinch of ground cinnamon (optional)

- ½ cup coconut or almond vegan yogurt
- 1 banana, sliced
- ½ cup sliced strawberries
- ½ cup sliced kiwi
- ¼ cup fresh blueberries

1. Preheat oven to 300 degrees F.

2. Place the tortilla on a baking sheet and brush lightly with the coconut oil. Drizzle with the maple syrup just enough to lightly sweeten the crust—too much will burn. Sprinkle with the cinnamon, if desired.

3. Toast the tortilla crust for 3–5 minutes; it should be crisp but not burnt. Let the tortilla cool.

4. Spread a thin layer of the yogurt over the crust and arrange the sliced fruit in an alternating pattern to your liking. Serve immediately.

Serves 2.

Potassium Punch Smoothie

This is great when you need a quick and easy dessert. It also doubles as a terrific breakfast smoothie, loaded with potassium, magnesium, and protein. It will keep you energized and satisfied throughout your morning.

- 1 banana (the riper the better)
- ¼ cup fresh blueberries
- ⅓ cup fresh strawberries, hulled
- ½ cup vegan almond butter
- 1 cup coconut milk

1. Combine all of the ingredients in a blender and blend on low speed until smooth. You can add ice if you desire a thicker shake.

Serves 2.

Bountiful Bread Pudding

Bread pudding may be the quintessential comfort food when it comes to desserts. Although you want to limit your intake of flour-based products, this recipe is great for those times when you do want to indulge just a little.

- ½ cup coconut oil, at room temperature, plus additional for greasing pan
- ¼ cup coconut milk
- 3 tablespoons pure maple syrup, plus additional for drizzling
- 3 tablespoons flaxseed mixed with 9 tablespoons water
- 12 slices whole wheat bread, cut into ½-inch pieces
- 1 (8-ounce) can crushed pineapple, with liquid
- ½ cup raisins

1. Preheat the oven to 350 degrees F. Grease a baking dish lightly with coconut oil and set aside.

2. In a medium saucepan over low heat, combine the coconut milk and maple syrup, and cook just until the syrup is completely dissolved in the milk.

3. Transfer the milk mixture to a large bowl and whisk in the flaxseed-water mixture. Stir in the bread, pineapple, raisins, and coconut oil. Stir until the bread is well soaked.

4. Transfer the mixture to the prepared baking dish and bake for about 40 minutes, or until the bread pudding is firm and fluffy. Drizzle with maple syrup before serving.

Serves 8.

French Toast à la Mode

The name is enough to make your mouth water, but the aroma of this dish when it's cooking can seduce from miles away. This is wonderful as either a dessert or a sweet breakfast treat. Use very ripe bananas to get the best flavor from this dish.

- 3 ripe bananas, pureed
- 2 cups coconut milk
- 2 teaspoons coconut oil
- 6 slices whole wheat bread
- 1 quart vegan ice cream (rice, almond, and coconut are all good choices)
- Pure maple syrup (optional)

1. Place the pureed bananas on a rimmed plate and pour the coconut milk in a shallow medium bowl.

2. In a large skillet over medium heat, heat the coconut oil until quite hot.

3. Dip each slice of bread completely in the banana puree and then completely in the coconut milk. Add each slice of bread to the pan and brown on both sides.

4. Transfer each cooked slice to a plate, top with a small scoop of ice cream, and drizzle with maple syrup, if desired.

Serves 6.

Easy Peach Cobbler

This recipe is great for when you need something sweet but you need it in a hurry and without a lot of fuss. Use peaches that are perfectly ripe, if not a bit overripe, for the best flavor.

- ¼ cup coconut oil
- 8 peaches, sliced
- ½ cup whole wheat flour
- ½ cup coconut milk
- ⅓ cup pure maple syrup, plus additional for drizzling
- 2 tablespoons ground cinnamon, plus additional for sprinkling
- 1 teaspoon baking powder

1. Preheat oven to 375 degrees F.

2. Melt the coconut oil in the bottom of a baking dish by placing it briefly in the oven. Add the sliced peaches to the dish and set aside.

3. In a medium bowl, combine the flour, coconut milk, maple syrup, cinnamon, and baking powder and mix well. Add the mixture to the peaches and stir well to coat.

4. Bake the cobbler for 40 minutes.

5. While it cools, drizzle the top with maple syrup and sprinkle with cinnamon.

Serves 6.

CONCLUSION: WRAPPING IT UP

The China Study did more than just prove that a diet free from processed foods and meat is good for you; it proved that it can literally heal disease and keep your body and your mind functioning optimally. One of the best things about the diet is that it isn't a diet at all. Rather, it's a prescription for better living. There are no hard-and-fast rules nor is there an ideology behind it that dictates morality or perfection.

The idea, supported by decades of research, is that the closer your diet is to be composed of 100 percent whole, natural foods completely free from animal products, processing, and chemicals, the healthier you will be. Even a 10-percent reduction in consumption of those foods can produce significant results. Completely eliminating them will turn your life around.

Some people find it easier to incorporate some processed or commercially prepared foods into their daily life. Foods such as organic whole grain breads and pastas, as well some sauces or other items prepared with minimal additives and handling are fine. The key is to look at your labels. If it has ingredients in it that you can't pronounce, it's probably best to skip it. Watch the sodium content, too, because many processed foods are high in salt.

Another food that many people in the China Study ate either somewhat regularly or on a limited basis is fish. Though it is a meat product, the fatty acids in fish are good for you. Still, the people who were the healthiest were those who abstained from all meat products completely. Allowing meat on "special occasions" can be a slippery slope that leads to more and more "special occasions." So if you're serious about eliminating animal products, it may be best to just commit all the way.

We hope that you found this book about the China Study Diet helpful and informative. Enjoy the recipes and use them as a basis to create your own delicious healthy meals and snacks. You'll soon find that it's just as easy and satisfying to eat foods that are good for you as it is to eat foods that aren't, so at least give it a try. Your body will thank you for it.

We wish you happy and healthful living.

GLOSSARY

amino acids—the chief components of proteins, they are synthesized by the body or obtained through food, and they are essential to good health. The human body can make all but eight of the essential amino acids; the remaining eight must be obtained through diet, either by eating animal products (less healthful) or by eating a wide variety of plants, nuts, and legumes (very healthful).

antioxidants—substances that inhibit oxidation or the reactions of free radicals. Antioxidants can be found in abundance in fruits and vegetables, and they help prevent aging.

atherosclerosis—a degenerative disease of the arteries in which the arteries are thickened by abnormal fatty deposits. Atherosclerosis can lead to heart disease.

autoimmune diseases—any disease in which the body attacks its own molecules, cells, or organs. Autoimmune diseases can be triggered in a variety of ways, including poor diet choices, and can be helped by proper nutrition, such as eating a plant-based diet.

China Study—the most comprehensive, longest-running health and nutrition study in medical history. Conducted by T. Colin Campbell, PhD, jointly with Cornell University and the Chinese Academy of

Preventive Medicine, the study proves that diseases of affluence are virtually nonexistent in those who eat a plant-based diet.

diseases of affluence—diseases such as Alzheimer's, diabetes, osteoporosis, and heart disease that afflict prosperous societies that have adopted less-than-healthful eating and lifestyle habits.

free radicals—cells that have become unstable due to a lost ion, and as a result, they can damage cells, proteins, and DNA by altering their chemical structure. Aging is directly related to the damage free radicals inflict upon the body. Fortunately, free radicals are inhibited and, in some cases, neutralized by antioxidants found in fruits and vegetables.

genetic predisposition—when used specifically in relationship to diseases, it refers to a marker or characteristic in the DNA that makes it possible for certain diseases to be activated. However, genetic predisposition for a disease—cancer, diabetes, heart disease—means only that the predisposition exists, not that it is inevitable; it can be activated only by the right (or in this case, wrong) environmental or dietary trigger.

HDL cholesterol—(good cholesterol) these high-density lipoproteins remove bad cholesterol from the bloodstream, helping to maintain healthy arteries and blood flow. By eating a mostly plant-based diet, you can assist your body in lowering your LDL levels and maintaining healthful HDL levels.

LDL cholesterol—(bad cholesterol) these low-density lipoproteins can leave deposits in the arteries, leading to atherosclerosis and heart disease. High LDL levels have been linked to a diet high in animal products and unsaturated fats.

saturated fat—fats whose chains of carbon atoms hold as many hydrogen atoms as possible; in other words, the chains are saturated with hydrogen. Saturated fats are unhealthful and can be found in animal products and fried foods.

trans fats—man-made fat created by the hydrogenation of vegetable oils that makes oils more shelf-stable. Because they are a foreign substance not found in nature, your body doesn't know what to do with them, and they cause clogged arteries that lead to heart disease and stroke.

type 3 diabetes—the new classification of Alzheimer's disease, which is the result of the resistance to insulin in the brain. A diet full of simple sugars and starches exacerbate diabetes by causing spikes in insulin and eventually creating insulin resistance. To counteract type 3 diabetes and diabetes of all kinds, consume complex carbohydrates like those found in plants, which release glucose at healthful rates and trigger slow, natural releases of insulin.

unsaturated fats—fats whose chains of carbon atoms hold fewer hydrogen atoms, such as polyunsaturated fats and monounsaturated fats. These healthful fats can be found in many plants, including olive oil, almonds, and avocados.

INDEX

CPSIA information can be obtained at www.ICGtesting.com
Printed in the USA
LVOW06s0140161113

361446LV00001B/3/P

9 781623 152055